MW01463188

To Katy,
Hope you enjoy this tale—
Ellen Gusheon

THE
HYDRANGEA
PE✡PLE

THE HYDRANGEA PEOPLE

A NOVEL

CHARLES GERSHON

Mose Cade Books
Asheville, North Carolina

Copyright © 2002 by Charles Gershon

All rights reserved, including the right of reproduction in whole or in part in any form.

Requests for permission to make copies of any part of the work should be mailed to the following address:

Mose Cade Books
20 Battery Park Avenue
Suite 609
Asheville, NC 28801

Printed in the United States of America

ISBN: 0-9725419-1-8

Text set in ITC Giovanni and Trajan
Cover and interior designed by Robert Mott for
Robert Mott & Associates, Keswick, VA

Printed in the United States of America

First edition 2002

AUTHOR'S NOTE

This is a work of fiction. Any relationship between reality and this book is coincidental.

ACKNOWLEDGEMENTS

There are many people who helped me write this book.

Jeffrey Cohn, M.D. of Birmingham, Alabama spent an evening with me talking about my amorphous idea for a book. He had a story to tell, and he told it well. Later, Jeffrey read a very rough first draft of the manuscript and offered his usual scholarly critique.

Morris Abrams (of blessed memory) helped me understand daily life for Jews in Eastern Europe during the Holocaust. Simon Fraley (of blessed memory) told me stories of his adventures as a partisan fighting with the Russian army in WWII and translated many passages into Yiddish.

Louis Schmier, Professor of History at Valdosta State University, welcomed me into his house and filled my notebooks with stories of Jewish people in small Southern towns. He originated the hydrangea people concept.

Cathy Hauck and Alexa Selph took a blue pen to the manuscript and sharpened an unmanageable bunch of pages into something that made sense.

Doug Kessler, Richard Bernstein, Trudy Reynolds, Susan Tourial, and Pano Lamis read the next version of the book and offered valuable insight and encouragement.

Over many bowls of oatmeal at the Landmark Diner, Jud Knight and I talked about the craft of writing. Jud is a great writer, and I will forever be grateful for his advice to stay on the spine of the book and leave out the parts people won't read.

Karen Risch did a great job helping me turn the final manuscript into the book in your hands.

Deidre Knight of the Knight Agency is the best agent any writer can have.

Jackie and Lamar Perlis of Cordele, Georgia opened up their house to my family and told me all about the Jewish history of Cordele. They took us to services at the Fitzgerald Hebrew Congregation, which was one of the highlights of working on this book. The members of the congregation inspired me to continue this project when it appeared I had reached a dead end. Jackie and Lamar are responsible for one of the main characters in this book, Buddy Ambrose.

The staff at the United States Holocaust Memorial Museum helped with research on Displaced-Persons Camps and the British blockade of Palestine.

Last but certainly not least, there is well-known Atlanta writer, Robert Coram. Without Robert, I would never have had the courage to write this book. Robert, you are truly a friend in fact and fiction.

DEDICATION

To Lynette, Alex, and Katie.

*To the many Frieda and Nathan Lanskys of America.
You have enriched every community
in which you have lived.*

She steps out of line to the left,
and her father to the right.
One side's a cold clean death,
the other is an endless night.

—Janis Ian, "Tattoo"

All that is necessary for the triumph of evil
is that good men do nothing.

—Edmund Burke

PROLOGUE

THE DAY I WAS BORN, IT RAINED. In Atlanta, it was a soft, lilting, sweet rain that gently massaged the hood of my anorak while we walked toward her home. Out of the corner of my eye, I watched her zip her coat and wondered if I could really see my reflection in her face. She wanted me to stay with her and talk more, but I wouldn't. Maybe if I had, she would have told me this nightmare was only a dream. But it wasn't a dream, because it was true, and there was no way for her to tell me anything different.

As I left her home, the rain washed along the windows of my car as if a collector were gently cleaning his prized roadster. The rain poured down on the woman, matting her beautiful blond hair, but, undeterred, she waved goodbye to me with the cadence of the wipers. She had a look of fulfillment on her face—as well she should, for she had been searching for completeness and had found it. I had thought I was complete, but now my search had just begun. What a difference! Of course, it doesn't matter, because reality becomes an illusion when the fantasy is exposed.

On the way to Cordele, it continued to rain. First this way then that, the rain poured in sheets just as it always does in this outpost of southern Georgia. Funny how it rains down here. It's like throwing a bucket of water in the face of a man dying of thirst: Sure, he needs the water, but not all at once. I have walked over parched peanut fields, only hours after a heavy rain, wondering if the sandy soil was really cheesecloth.

As I drive *home*—what a strange word!—to confront my parents, I'm not sure how any of this will turn out. Okay, *confront* may be too strong, and *discuss* too formal, but certainly *ask* is inadequate. But, that is what I must do—ask my parents to tell me the woman was lying. Of course, she wasn't lying, and they won't be able to tell me she was. Sure, they'll cough, clear their throats, hem and haw, furrow their brows, rub their tired old hands. But they never lie, and they won't be able to now.

Maybe I shouldn't even mention it to them. After all, they have breathed into me a life that has been far better than I ever could have expected, and infinitely richer and more rewarding than I have deserved. But I have to tell them I know their secret. Our secret, now.

I look up from the monotonous rhythm of the wipers and stare at my image in the rearview mirror. I see myself as I never have: a bit player in my own life's story and the only actor in the play who hasn't known the plot.

—From the Diary of Sammy Lansky

CHAPTER ONE 1

DAMN GOOD THING SAMMY NEVER CLEANED HIS DESK. He would have knocked himself out for sure when his head hit it, had it not been full of papers, charts, and doctor's magazines. Exhausted, he tried to open his eyes, but the lids weighed a ton apiece, so he gave in to the rack monster and slobbered all over *The Journal of Urology* and Gertrude Tinsley's chart.

Suddenly he bolted awake and out of his seat as if he'd been poked with a cattle prod. His assistant, Mary Ponder, was outside assaulting the door like it had personally pissed her off and she was getting even.

Bam! Bam! Boom! Mary hit the door hard. "You in there, Dr. Lansky?" *Bam! Bam!* "You in there?"

Sammy didn't dare open the door, because he thought she might knock it on top of him.

"Come in! Come in!" he yelled, loud enough for everyone three floors above and below the office to hear him.

Mary, a sturdy country girl reared on red-eye gravy and ham biscuits, marched in. She believed right and wrong had been determined two thousand years before and were immutable, just as sure as the sun rose in the sky in the morning and the moon showed up at night.

"Dr. L., don't forget the big meeting tonight at the Rich Carlton," Mary prompted him as she checked her clipboard for other notes. She found a few and put them on Sammy's desk.

"Would that be the *Ritz* Carlton, May-ree?" Sammy was an educated man—undergraduate engineering at Georgia Tech, medical school at Emory—but practicing his Southernese with pronunciations like "May-ree" kept him grounded, and to tell the truth, he loved reminding people he had made it to the top of the mountain from the small town of Cordele, Georgia.

"I guess," Mary said, checking her notes one last time. "Let's see . . . think that's about it. Good night, Dr. L." She placed the clipboard under her arm and marched out, loosening the hinges of the door as she slammed it closed.

Sammy fumbled through the papers on his desk, then opened his top drawer and, after searching for a minute, found the engraved invitation to that night's soiree:

> *The Georgia Stone Institute*
> *In celebration of its first year*
> *Cordially invites you to a dinner*
> *At the Ritz Carlton, Buckhead*
> *April 9, 1986*
> *Cocktails 6:30 P.M.*
> *Dinner 7:30 P.M.*
> *RSVP by April 6, 1986*

He stretched out in his office chair and smiled. Invitation in hand, he walked to the bank of windows as dusk settled over the city and looked out over the majesty of Atlanta. What was it Henry Grady said a century ago? Something about raising a "brave new city." Well, here it was, a phoenix hoisted from the ashes of Sherman's march to the sea. Directly to the south, Sammy could see the most well-known memorial to the great journalist, the massive Grady Hospital, the county facility where taxpayer dollars, when not misappropriated, were used to care for pimps, whores, drug addicts, members of gun and knife clubs, and other downtrodden souls. Sammy stretched and smiled. *Just think. If it had been up to Rachel, I'd be at Grady right now serving humankind, making a difference. What a joke.*

He rubbed his fingers along the invitation and laughed out loud. *Yeah, what a joke.*

◆ ◆ ◆

COCKTAILS AND HORS D'OEUVRES WERE PRESENTED in a hall just outside the clubby room where dinner was to be served. Of the one hundred urologists who received invitations, ninety-eight showed up, and when Sammy arrived, they treated him like their grand poobah. The other urologists stood in line to shake his hand, and several of them seemed to have a hard time letting go. Thanks, Sammy. Great job, Sammy. How can we thank you enough, Sammy? On and on went the kissing up until Sammy thought he would wretch from the sickening sweetness.

Dellwood Dole, the businessman who had masterminded the whole venture, and his partner and attorney, Henry Morton, worked the room, thanking everyone for their support during the year. Finally, the gong signaled time to move into the main room. Dellwood and Henry went to the head table and, as they sat, Dellwood motioned for Sammy and his partner, Mo Gordon, to join them. Dinner was served, and when the desserts appeared, Dellwood rose and tapped his glass. He was small, thin, and (in his own words) elegant. Dellwood's parents should have named him Dandy, for the shoe certainly fit. He never met a mirror he didn't like, particularly when his image was in it. Though he was probably about five-seven, his female companions were always Amazons. As he began to speak, he stroked his full head of blond hair and moved his hands about as if directing the words flowing from his mouth.

"I'm so happy to tell all of you that, in addition to the professional fees you have collected thus far, we do have some profit from Georgia Stone to share with the members of your doctor's professional group, Lithotripsy Associates. You'll be getting a check in a day or two."

Sammy had a hard time looking at Dellwood, because he was sure he would begin to laugh uncontrollably. Dellwood acted as if he pulled words from his mouth and sprinkled them onto to the public like Tinkerbell's dust. But, over the top or not, the message was a good one, and loud cheers filled the room.

A urologist from Savannah got up, raised his glass, and shouted above the din, "To Dellwood Dole and Henry Morton for showing us how to make money in two places at the same time!"

"Cheers!" the crowd responded in unison.

"An' to Mo Gordon 'n' Sammy Lansky for having the foresight to make this a doctor-owned deal!" shouted an inebriated doctor whose colleagues helped him back into his seat.

The crowd was in a frenzy now, as frenzied as doctors can get, clapping and cheering and slapping each other on their backs. Mo Gordon, in his hand-tailored Mario Bosco suit, stood on a chair and took a deep bow.

Dellwood pulled Mo back into his seat and waved his red silk handkerchief to get everyone's attention. "I think another round of applause is due Sam and Mo for being willing to take care of patients who have been referred by their partners in Lithotripsy Associates. After all, without that sacrifice on their part, this would have been much more difficult. Sam, Mo," Dellwood said, motioning for them to rise. "Please stand and accept our deepest congratulations."

Sammy and Mo stood, but as Mo began to get back on the chair, Dellwood grabbed his arm and glowered at him. Mo got off the chair, bowed, then sat.

The celebration broke up at about eleven. After the last of the doctors stumbled out of the room, Dellwood put his arms around Mo's and Sammy's shoulders and said, "You boys had better wash your feet, because when the docs get their checks in the next day or so, they are going to be kissing them.

"Speaking of money," he continued, "let's find a quiet place where we can do some business."

Dellwood, Henry, Mo, and Sammy went to a table that had already been cleared. Dellwood motioned to the hotel staff that they were not to be disturbed.

"Well, gentlemen," Dellwood began with a smirk. "We've got some checks coming, as well. I took the liberty of bringing them instead of mailing them. I hope," he said with an impish look, "you don't mind." Dellwood handed an envelope to each board member.

Sammy noticed Mo and Henry put theirs away, so he did the same. There was some small talk and mention of another meeting, but Sammy paid little attention as he continued to finger the envelope he had just put in his inside pocket.

The four men walked out of the Ritz into a cool spring evening. Sammy kept rubbing the inside pocket of his coat to make sure the envelope hadn't flown away. *Small talk, small talk. When will it stop?* Sammy thought. It finally did, and the four men sauntered off to their respective cars. Sammy had been patient enough, so he tore open the envelope and removed a letter from the Georgia Stone Institute.

Dear Dr. Lansky:

We would like to thank you for your support of the lithotriptor. As a result of that support, we are now able to make a distribution according to your percentage of ownership.

You own <u>five</u> shares through your participation in Lithotripsy Associates of the Georgia Stone Institute. The check enclosed reflects your share of the profits for the <u>first nine months</u> of operation. Please keep in mind that collections run ninety days behind. Thus, even though we've been in operation for a full twelve months, we have collected for only nine.

Keep up the good work. If there are ever any questions, please do not hesitate to call.

Sincerely,

Dellwood Dole
LithoServices

The check was attached to the letter. The stub above it read:

Distribution of Profits
Gross: $940,000
Per share: $1,880 (500 shares)
Number of shares held: 5

He unfolded the check and saw it was drawn on the Chattahoochee Bank. The number in the small rectangle was $9,400. Sammy smiled smugly. A nice little lagniappe for his generous six-figure salary, and this was for only nine months! He turned on the ignition, put his car into reverse, moved back a few feet, then got the feeling there was more in the envelope—it wasn't empty. He moved the car back into the space and, with the engine still running, turned on the dome light and put his hand back in the envelope. There was another note.

> Dear Dr. Lansky,
> The amount contained herein represents your percentage of the distribution owed the general partner, LithoServices. Our bank is happy to serve your needs. Please see us at your earliest convenience to discuss dispersal of the assets contained herewith.
>
> Maxwell Cherry
> First Fulton Savings and Loan

Sammy unfolded the other check. When he saw the amount, he was stunned. The bottom line was $940,000!

He looked at the stub, his hands shaking.

> *Georgia Stone Institute*
> *Sammy Lansky, 25% (18.75 shares) = $940,000*

Ho-ly shit, Sammy thought. In a daze, he backed up his car again. He was rich. Beyond any unbridled dreams, beyond his wildest imagination—he was rich, filthy rich! Nine-hundred-forty-thousand dollars! Hell, that was for only nine months. For twelve months, it was . . . what? One third more—over $1.2 million. And he could expect that year after year for at least five years. Now he understood how Mo lived so well: Mo was involved in a bunch of similar deals with Dellwood.

He looked at his watch: 11:30 P.M. It was too late for a celebratory drink in the hotel bar, so he drove home in a daze. He had made a lot of money practicing urology with Mo, but this good fortune put him into another category. He had set goals for himself—the major one was to be wealthy. Tonight he had attained that goal.

Sammy arrived at his apartment and stood outside, shaking his head and laughing to himself. Here he was, a rich man still living in a dump. He and Rachel had arrived in Atlanta more than four years ago needing something affordable, so this garage apartment behind an old mansion in the silk stocking neighborhood of Druid Hills fit the bill. The upstairs consisted of a bedroom with a closet big enough for two winter coats and a claustrophobic bathroom with a claw-foot tub surrounded by a flowered plastic curtain. The toilet was so close to the vanity Sammy had to sit sideways so his legs didn't end up at his chin. The kitchenette had white metal cabinets and linoleum floors and appliances that belonged in a museum.

He entered, climbed the stairs, and headed toward the bedroom to tell Rachel the news. He found her sleeping soundly and decided to leave her alone. As quietly as he could, he threw ice into a glass, found a bottle of scotch in the liquor cabinet, and poured it. The pungent odor of the liquid filled his nostrils. He walked downstairs into his favorite room, the living room—"the hall of mirrors," as Rachel had dubbed it. The entire room was mirrored and, at one time, must have been a dance studio. He sat and took a long drink. Everywhere he looked he saw Sammy Lansky, a man who had the world by the short hairs.

He flashed back to twenty-five years before when he and a boyhood friend, Clete Towns, had been watching the trains pass through downtown Cordele. Clete, leaning against a tree, had waxed poetic on how life was all about timing and being in the right place at the right time. Sammy smiled when he thought now of his countrified philosopher friend.

"Call it fate, luck, timing, whatever the hell you want," Clete had said. "Success don't have nothing to do with intelligence, Sammy. It's got everything to do with putting your young self in a position to suc-ceed."

Sammy laughed to himself and took another long drink of the scotch. Clete had been right: By joining Mo in practice, Sammy had put himself in a position to, as Clete said, "suc-ceed." He had gone to medical school to make his parents proud of him, and they were. He had joined Mo to make money, and he had.

When he'd finished his residency at the University of Michigan, Rachel had wanted him to join the staff at Emory and Grady, but he'd known what that would mean—all prestige and no money—kind of like being a Polish count. His wife had been furious about Sammy's decision to join Mo.

"You don't know anything about that hospital where he practices," she'd warned him.

"Mo says it's fine. Busiest place on the south side of Atlanta."

"Yeah, well, Meridian Hospital near Ann Arbor was busy, too, and I'm sure those guys made a lot of money, but I wouldn't want to go there even if it was three days after I died."

They'd argued nonstop for months, and in the end, he had won. Within three months, he'd known he had done the right thing, because during that time, Mo had taught him how medicine equaled money. Mo periodically reviewed Sammy's charts, not for quality issues, but to make sure he got the most out of each procedure for billing. At first, Sammy had been irritated and intimidated by this supervision. But, when he'd seen how he could turn a simple $200 procedure into a $600 procedure just by coding it a certain way, he'd understood Mo's intentions, and now he was happy to have had the help.

"Forget all the ivory tower bullshit you learned in residency," Mo had told him. "Those professors are so busy being big shots that they don't know anything about the real world."

He'd put some billing records in front of Sammy. "Code 52281 is cysto," Mo had said. "We've already gone over that one. It's two hundred dollars. Code 52276, urethral dilatation, major—one hundred. Code 52224, fulguration of minor lesion—one hundred twenty-five. Code 52204, bladder biopsy—hundred bucks. Patients want to make sure there's no tumor. You can even do a cystogram, 51600. A simple X-ray of the bladder, a cystogram, adds a hundred bucks. Look at what you got. Same procedure, maybe fifteen minutes longer because of the X-ray, but instead of two hundred dollars, you got six hundred twenty-five dollars. According to the formula I got worked out, based on the number of patients you're seeing, you *should* be doing ten to fifteen cystos a week. Ten a week at six hundred is right at three hundred thousand in cystos alone."

Mo had said that when he put on his silk sport coat, got in his huge Mercedes sedan equipped with the finest stereo equipment, and drove to his six-thousand-square-foot home, he knew he had escaped his humble Brooklyn beginnings.

"Look, you and I are from the same background. My dad's a tailor. I say 'is' because at seventy-eight, he's still slaving away in his little shop in Brooklyn. My mom tells everyone he works because he loves it so much. Shit, he works because he's got no damn choice. He and Mama got this bad habit of wanting to eat. They sure as hell can't live on social security."

Sammy held the glass in front of his eyes and looked through it. The liquid smiled with him as it massaged his brain. Here in the hall of mirrors sat the king of the Lanskys. Never before in the history of the Lansky family, dating back at least to the time of the Crusades, had anyone risen to such heights. Never before had members of his family had one thing more than they needed. Poverty and pogroms, poverty and pogroms: That was all his ancestors had gotten generation after generation. He had come from nowhere, born in Europe after the war, the only child of Holocaust survivors, a Jewish boy reared in the vacuum of Cordele, Georgia. Yet he was sitting here tonight as a king. Long live the king!

CHAPTER TWO

SAMMY STAYED UP HALF THE NIGHT, so when he arose at 5:30, the only thing he was afraid of was that he might live. But, hangover or no, he was now King of the Lanskys, and today was the first day of his reign.

He showered, dressed, put the checks in his sport coat pocket, and tiptoed from the apartment, leaving Rachel sound asleep. He didn't have a surgical case until eleven, so he decided to make rounds then head straight to the bank before he rubbed the big check so much it disintegrated.

"Good morning, Dr. Lansky," called Beulah Campbell, the head nurse. She was a large, buxom, black woman who ran the urology floor at Gate City Medical Center as though it were her personal fiefdom. She was one of the few nurses who still wore a starched white cap with her nursing school pin prominently displayed on the front. All of her nurses wore white dresses; no pants were allowed. They referred to the physicians and surgeons on what she jokingly called a first-name basis. All of them had the same first name: Doctor.

"Hello, Mrs. Campbell. Is Dr. Tescione here yet?"

"Waiting for you in the back, I believe," the head nurse replied.

"Thanks." Sammy went into the coffee room, where he found Elizabeth Tescione, the intern assigned to urology, swapping love stories with one of the nurses. She must have heard someone enter the room, because she turned around slightly, revealing her more than ample bosom, which was outlined by her tight, black sweater.

"Hello, Samm—Dr. Lansky." She greeted him with a half-hearted smile. "How are you?"

"Fine," he said. He loved to watch her full, dark, Italian, kiss-me lips move as the words drifted out of her mouth. "Let's go," Sammy urged her. "I've got a busy day."

The early morning sun hit Sammy as they walked into a patient's room. Holding his right hand over his eyes, he went over to the window and closed the blinds. "Ah, much better," he said. He looked at the bed—the covers were thrown back, and the bed was empty.

"Mr. Palkowski has escaped," Sammy noted dryly, glancing sideways at Elizabeth.

The sound of a gloriously long fart emanated from the bathroom.

"Close the windows, Libby." A broad smile creased Sammy's face. "Canadian geese a thousand miles away heard that mating call."

The bathroom door opened, and a little man appeared.

"Those suppositories are just like you said, Dr. Lansky," the little man reported in a European accent. He straightened the back of his gown and waddled toward the bed. "They are gifts from the gods."

"Great. Now lie down and let me examine you, Kasper." Sammy pointed to the bed, and the old man hobbled in that direction and farted again as he lay down.

"Ahh . . . ohh. . . ," he said as he positioned himself.

"Any path back, Libby?" Sammy asked, referring to the microscopic analysis of tissue.

She had asked him to call her Elizabeth, and she winced every time he didn't. "His pathology showed the tumor to be contained within the renal pelvis." She looked at the chart as she spoke. "With no evidence of neoplasm in the ureter or bladder," she finished and put the chart down on the bed.

Sammy shook the patient's hand and held it as he spoke. "Looks like you're gonna have to find some other way to die, Kasper. We cured you of this here tumor."

"Ahh . . ." Kasper moved up in bed and, still shaking Sammy's hand, smiled. "Wonderful, wonderful," he said. Tears rose in his eyes. "You are a great man, doctor, and my family and I will never forget you." He turned toward the intern. "You either, dear."

Sammy looked at Elizabeth as he smiled. Her cold look said she would prefer *doctor* to *dear*.

"Let's get his drain out today," Sammy instructed. "I think he'll be ready to go home in three or four days."

She nodded and wrote on her pad.

They walked into the next room, where Shorty Anderson, dying of incurable prostate cancer, was wasting away. The stale, quiet air of life's conclusion filled the room. Sammy had admitted him for pain management because Shorty's family could no longer take care of him at home. Plans to move him to a hospice had been canceled. The next move—certainly within forty-eight hours—would be to Patterson's Funeral Home.

"Hi, Dr. Lansky." Shorty's frail wife addressed him in a barely audible voice.

"How'd he do last night?" Sammy asked. "Did he rest okay?"

Mrs. Anderson shook her head and looked at the floor. Sammy patted her shoulder and sat down on the patient's bed. Shorty was awake but obviously in a twilight state.

"Any luck on yesterday's question?" Sammy took the patient's hand in his. Shorty barely opened his eyes and shook his head.

"It was Wes Covington," Sammy told him.

The patient smiled and whispered, "That's right. Bruton was in center, not left."

Every day, Sammy asked Shorty a baseball trivia question. The rule was simple: Shorty could get no outside help; he had to sink or swim on his own. Yesterday's question was who had played left field for the 1958 Milwaukee Braves.

Sammy squeezed the patient's hand. He asked, "You ready for tomorrow's question?"

A glimmer of brightness peaked from the hollow depths of Shorty's eyes, like a star's light barely visible from a distant galaxy. "Sure, Doc. Shoot."

"The year Maris hit sixty-one homers, there were two Yankee outfielders on that team who eventually made it to the Hall of Fame. Who were they?" Sammy asked.

"Tough one," rasped the patient. "Got to think about it. Tell you tomorrow."

Sammy rose, winked at Mrs. Anderson, who smiled, then he said, "That's such a tough one, I'll give you two days."

Shorty waved, closed his eyes, and drifted off to sleep.

As they exited the room, Sammy's intern had a quizzical look on her face. "Mantle was one of them. Who was the other?" she asked.

"Damn impressive, Tescione," Sammy said, patting her on the back. "Yogi Berra," he answered as they walked down the hall.

The next room was at the end of the hall. Again the sun shone in their faces as they entered. "Wow, everyone wants to see Stone Mountain this morning, I guess," Sammy said as he walked over to let the blinds down. The patient, Durwood Black, was in the bathroom, shaving. "How you doing, Mr. Black? Seems like you're ready to leave."

"Yep, I'm ready to roll," the patient said, pointing to his packed bags. "Soon as Loretta gets here, that is."

"Well, c'mon. Sit down, and let me examine you." Sammy motioned for the patient to sit on the bed. Durwood, still in his hospital gown, sat down on the side of the bed.

Sammy examined the patient's side and nodded his approval. "Looks good, Durwood," he said. "Not too much bruising."

"Yeah, Dr. Lansky. This here lithotripsy was a whole lot easier than that there procedure my cousin had a coupla years ago. You know the one I told you about, where they made a hole inside his kidney to get the stone out? I mean to tell you, he had blood and corruption draining out of him for weeks. He was in a hell of a mess. I mean, I went down to Conyers to visit him, and he could barely—"

"The doctor's busy, Durwood," said the patient's wife as she entered the room. "Let him do the talking so we can get out of here some time today."

"I was just telling him—," he said before Loretta grabbed his arm and squeezed.

Sammy smiled. "Glad everything went so well. Now, remember what I told you about having to pass all the stone particles. They're going to look just like sand, and you've got to strain through a wire mesh so we can see how much you pass and send some of the material off for analysis. Okay?"

Durwood began again. "Yeah, my cousin did that, but I got no idea how them doctors figured out what was corruption and what was stone. They must've . . ." By now, his wife's fingernails were dug so deeply into the meat of his hand he looked as if he was going to pass out as he stopped talking.

The woman nodded and, still holding her husband in a death grip, she shook hands with Sammy.

"The nurses will give you a sheet of instructions," Sammy said, pulling a prescription pad out of his coat pocket. "Here's a prescription for pain pills." He wrote on the pad and handed a piece of paper to the Blacks.

"I'll see you in two weeks," Sammy said.

He and the intern left the room. "See you in the O.R. at eleven, Libb—Elizabeth. I've got to go. Let me know if you need anything."

♦ ♦ ♦

HE DEPOSITED THE SMALLER CHECK IN HIS BANK, then drove to First Fulton Savings and Loan. It was a beautiful spring morning, and as he got out of his car and sauntered across the parking lot toward the small but impressive building, a slight breeze blew in his face. The inside was well appointed and as quiet as a library. Across from the tellers, he saw an attractive woman talking on the phone. Her nameplate said she was Anne Murnane.

When he approached her, she motioned for him to sit but continued to talk. Finally, she hung up, smiled at Sammy, and said, "May I help you, sir?"

Sammy rubbed the remaining check in his pocket, leaned forward and said, "Um, I need to see Mr. . . ." He pulled the letter out of his pocket, then continued, "Mr. Maxwell Cherry."

Without hesitation, Ms. Murnane spoke into the intercom on her desk, "Mr. Cherry, there's a—" She stopped and looked at Sammy. "Excuse me, what did you say your name is, sir?'

"Lansky," he replied. "Sammy Lansky."

She hit the button on the intercom again, and said, "Mr. Lansky is here to see you."

"Please send him in, Ms. Murnane."

Sammy thanked her and went into Cherry's glass-partitioned office.

"Hello, I'm Maxwell Cherry," he said, extending his hand to shake Sammy's then close the door. "Nice to meet you." Maxwell offered Sammy a seat.

He was a rotund man of medium height with thinning, dark hair that he slicked back. He had on an expensive suit garnished with a white pocket square and alligator suspenders. Sammy noticed his right cuff was monogrammed.

"Sammy Lansky. Nice to meet you, Mr. Cherry." Sammy situated himself on a small couch.

"Mr.—uh, Dr. Lansky. Would you like some coffee?"

Sammy nodded. Maxwell leaned toward the intercom and asked Anne for two cups. "How do you like it, doctor?" the banker asked, his finger still on the intercom button.

"Just sugar," Sammy replied.

After the coffee was served and the door closed, Maxwell spoke. "Mr. Dole has arranged for you to have a sweep account."

Sammy moved around in his seat. "What's a sweep account?"

"It means funds you put in are automatically swept into an interest-bearing account. We suggest opening several of these to keep each one under the federal insurance level." Maxwell took a sip of coffee then put his cup down and folded his hands on the desk. "We can also put you in touch with someone who'll help you invest the funds in the capital markets, if you'd like."

"Sounds okay to me," Sammy said, rubbing the check in his inside pocket. "I'd, uh, kind of like to make a deposit now if I could. It makes me, you know, a little nervous walking around with a check this size."

"I understand." Maxwell smiled, and his full, ruddy face and white teeth made him look cherubic. "If you'd sign some papers, we can arrange for the funds to be transferred to several money market accounts right now. Of course, your money will always be accessible to you. You'll receive some checks in the next few weeks."

Sammy agreed and signed his name twice on the three-page document, which he did not read. The banker's assistant sashayed into the office, took the papers, and asked Sammy for the check. He took it out of his pocket, hesitated for a moment, then handed it to her.

"Hmm," Sammy said, rising to leave. "Is that all?"

"Yes. Thanks, doctor." Maxwell rose, too, and extended his hand. "I'm sure we'll have a long, happy relationship."

Sammy walked slowly out of the bank, like someone who had forgotten to do or say something important. As he started to get into his car, he spotted Mo's Mercedes pulling into the parking lot. Sammy walked over and propped his arms on top of Mo's car.

"Hi, Mo," he called as his mentor opened the car door.

"Good to see you." Mo got out of his car. "Depositing your check?"

"Yeah, got here as soon as I could this morning," Sammy told him, reaching into his own car to retrieve sunglasses from the dashboard. "This bank's okay, isn't it? I mean, uh, you know, it's only got, what, two branches?"

"Solid as a rock." Mo bent down to check his appearance in the driver's side mirror. "Lots of personal service."

"Okay," Sammy said softly and without conviction. "Guess I'd better get to work."

Sammy got in his car, put the key in the ignition and reached for the door. He could smell his friend's strong cologne and realized that Mo was holding his door open. Sammy looked up at him.

"Sammy, this stone thing . . ." Mo adjusted his sunglasses. "It's going much better than anyone thought. I, uh, think we ought to keep the finances, you know, kind of quiet." Mo cleared his throat.

"I wouldn't . . . I mean, don't tell anyone how much we've made so far. You know that old saying: Loose lips sink ships. We've got a chance to make a lot of money on this thing. Too much talk and bragging might, you know . . . " Mo shrugged his shoulders. "It might, uh, upset things. Hospitals and insurance companies aren't used to us making this kind of money."

Sammy put his index finger to his mouth. "Mo, my lips are sealed."

"Good boy, Sammy," Mo said, slapping him on the back. "Good boy."

Later that day, outside the doctors' lounge, Sammy bumped into a fellow urologist, Jeffrey Kagan. "Hi, Jeff, what's going on?" Sammy asked in a soft voice.

"Just got my check from the lithotriptor." They walked together toward the professional building. Jeff continued, "Wish I'd bought the max number of shares. Damn thing is a cash cow. I only bought two shares, but, hell, I already doubled my money—put in two grand, made four. What a deal! Never heard of a return like that. Hundred percent return in less than a year." He paused by the door to the stairwell. "We owe you and Mo a helluva lot for putting the whole thing together. Y'all did a great job. It's about time docs started cashing in on things like this. Hospitals have been doing it for years."

"I think it's only gonna get better, Jeff." Sammy looked down at his beeping pager. "The insurance companies might cut down what they pay us, but by the time they do, we'll have paid off the machine. Our overhead will drop when compensation drops. I'd say we're in the driver's seat."

"Yeah, the only thing that worries me," Jeff said, looking around and lowering his voice, "is that some of our colleagues might start bragging about this kind of return. We probably ought to keep quiet about our windfall."

Sammy walked over to a house phone to answer his page. His colleague followed. "I completely agree, Jeff. This is too good a gold mine to ruin it."

"Boy, is that true." Jeff smiled as he started up the steps.

◆ ◆ ◆

"RACH, I'M HOME."

"Jeez, Sammy, another late one. What time did you get home last night? This machine has taken over your whole life."

Sammy climbed the stairs, entered the kitchen, and saw Rachel preparing dinner in jeans and a T-shirt. He kissed her on the cheek, then stood at her side, admiring his wife of almost thirteen years. She was tall and thin and, though now thirty-six, still had the smooth, ivory skin and jet black hair of a China doll.

"Sit down and let's have a glass of this." Sammy removed a bottle of cheap champagne from a brown paper bag.

"What's the occasion?" she asked as she sat. "Become a full partner today?"

"Nope, better than that."

Sammy went to a cabinet and withdrew two champagne glasses, which had *In Honor of the Wedding of Marla and Irvin, December 17, 1980* etched on each.

"Have a glass of the bubbly, Rach."

Rachel rose and exchanged their glasses for different ones, which she handed to Sammy. "At least use decent glasses. Marla and Irvin got divorced over a year ago."

Sammy smiled, poured two glasses of champagne, then pulled the check stubs from his pocket and handed them to Rachel as he sat down. She took a sip, then put her glass on the table and studied the figures.

"What're these checks? Where'd you get them?"

"Found them," he said with a smile, taking a large gulp of the liquid. "Was walking down the street yesterday, and they fell right out of the sky, kind of like manna from heaven." He looked upward as he spoke and kissed the side of his glass.

Rachel glared at Sammy, then looked back at the stubs. "Who gave you these checks?"

"The president of the United States gave them to me for being such a model citizen and proving that the immigration policy of this country has been a tremendous success." Sammy finished his champagne, stood, and moved the bottle from the counter top to the table. He poured himself another glass and offered more to Rachel, but she covered her glass. Raising his own, he said, "In fact, when Ronnie handed it to me, he called me a credit to my race."

Rachel showed no emotion as she looked up at Sammy then down at the stubs again. "Seriously, where'd you get these?"

"I earned them. Been working my butt off for over a year. Actually, longer than that. Hell!" he yelled as he slapped his hand against the table. "Everyone knew the lithotriptor was coming. Did they do anything about it? Shit, no. I'm the one who went to Munich for two boring weeks to study the machine. I'm the one who sucked up to the damn Germans so they'd remember us when the time came to hand out machines. I got the ball rolling here by getting Mo, Morton, and Dole involved. I deserve every damn dime I get." He hesitated for a moment as he took another sip of champagne. "You ought to be jumping for joy."

Without taking her eyes off the check stubs, Rachel slowly sipped the champagne. "Sammy, what does all this mean? Why the different amounts? Different banks?"

"Easy," he said, throwing his hands up in the air. "One's for my part as a doctor owning the lithotriptor. The other is for my position on the board of directors and being part of the administration of the machine."

She held one of the stubs in each hand and stared at him. "Which one's which? One stub says you own . . . let's see . . . five shares. The other one says eighteen and some change. I'm confused." She rose and leaned across the table, showing Sammy the papers. "I mean, are they paying you nearly a million dollars to sit on some board?"

"Hell, the board put the whole damn thing together. Some hospital would be making all the money if it had been left to the urologists in this state." He stood and took a swig of champagne. "The docs are lucky we did all the legwork. Shit, they're making a helluva lot more than they would've if they didn't own the thing. They ought to be kissing our asses."

He refilled his glass and leaned against the kitchen counter. "Look, how many times have I gotten home at eleven o'clock or midnight, tired as hell from blasting stones? While I've been doing that, some urologist in Savannah's having dinner at a nice restaurant or maybe even banging his wife. And guess who's being paid for my services? Not ol' Sammy 'The Slave' Lansky. No, the guy in Savannah is." He swallowed the whole glass of champagne and glared at his wife. "So I deserve the money. I earned it."

Rachel turned her palms toward him, signaling for Sammy to calm down. "Okay. Okay. I'll admit you've worked hard from the beginning. I don't pretend to understand this arrangement you guys have, but that's okay." She motioned for Sammy to sit, which he did, then she continued in a soft voice.

"But . . ." She hesitated for a second. "You've done nothing to earn a million bucks."

Sammy leaned across the table. "This is the eighties! Wealth is being created on a scale never seen before. Guys who made twenty grand a year as runners in brokerage houses are now making ten times that as financial consultants." He stopped to sit down. "Hell, the sky's the limit. That big boy of a check is for only nine months, and that's just the beginning. We've just signed up twenty-five more urologists. That brings us up to one hundred twenty-five and growing. Soon we'll be treating patients all day Saturday. Dole says I could easily make a million and a half a year, plus my share in the doctors' corporation on top of my salary."

Rachel stood and put the stubs squarely in front of Sammy. "So why are these checks drawn on two different banks?"

He shrugged. "Don't know. Mo says First Fulton is strong on personal service. Might be some business acquaintance of Dellwood Dole."

Rachel rubbed her forehead. "No one makes this kind of money in nine months," she said, shaking her head. "Something's wrong. I'm amazed that someone as smart as you didn't question the amounts."

Sammy jumped up and threw his glass against the ancient refrigerator. "Goddammit! Why the hell do you have to be so damn negative?" He slammed his fist on the table, pushing it enough to knock Rachel into her seat. "Once, just once in your life, try to look at the glass as half-full instead of half-empty. This is some good shit that's happened. Try to enjoy it." He fell into his chair and slumped.

Rachel, tears welling in her eyes, shook her head and spoke in a quiet voice. "Enjoy what, Sammy? The fact that you're never home? The fact that you've suddenly got all this money but can't really explain where it came from? Tell me what I'm supposed to be so happy about."

Sammy jumped out of his chair, throwing his arms open and knocking the champagne bottle off the table as he did. He picked it up and poured the remains in his glass. "Oh, excuse me, I forgot. I'm talking to Rachel Dziewinski of the infamous Fitzgerald Dziewinskis. Life is horrible, and only death brings peace."

Rachel's right hand slapped the side of Sammy's face as soon as he finished talking. He was pushed into his seat by the force and suddenness of her attack. With two steps, she stood over him, her eyes bulging, her chest heaving, her nostrils flaring.

"How your parents got you for a son is a mystery to me. The Almighty collected all their bad traits and stuffed them inside you." Rachel was shaking and was so close to Sammy that she spat on him as she spoke. "My parents had a right to be the way they were. How do you think you'd feel if you saw your little daughters raped and sodomized right in front of your eyes? Brutally defiled by some jackbooted subhumans who laughed the whole time!" Her voice had escalated to a yell, and she grabbed him by the collar.

"Two beautiful little girls screaming in Yiddish—'*Foter! Foter! Mameh! Mameh!*'—blood pouring from their delicate little bodies until, finally, the Nazi bastards gave them peace by slitting their throats."

She squeezed his collar as tightly as she could and stared into his eyes. He turned his head to avoid her glare. Slowly, she backed away from him, but her eyes, now dry and cold, never lost sight of his face. "Yeah, Sammy, sometimes only death brings peace."

Sammy stared straight ahead in silence. Rachel had a distant, empty gaze for about ten seconds. Her eyes were wide open, her mouth tightly closed. She went into the bedroom and returned a few seconds later with a piece of paper. She threw it across the table, giving Sammy a few seconds to look it over while she stood across from him.

He opened his hands in a pleading fashion, and said in a diminutive voice. "What, what's this got to do. . . ?"

Rachel leaned across the table and pointed at the paper. "This is the invitation to Mo and Sylvia's party tomorrow night." She leaned a little farther toward Sammy. "All of your business buddies will be there, and you're going to find out about these checks tomorrow night."

Sammy looked at the invitation again, then squirmed in his seat. "But . . . I mean, at a party . . . it . . . I mean, it may not be in the best of taste. I . . ."

She slammed her fist on the table, then smiled wryly. "Mo and his wife are so crude, they wouldn't know the difference."

Sammy sat up. "Wait a minute!" he screamed, then lowered his voice. "You know, I really like Mo."

She crossed her arms and smiled. "Tell you what. When we get home from the Gordons' party, I'm going to ask you a very simple question, which, I might add—" She moved across the room and got face to face with him again before continuing, "requires a very simple answer: Where did the $940,000 come from? You, Sammy Lansky, had better have that simple answer." She turned, walked into the bedroom, and slammed the door.

CHAPTER THREE 3

SAMMY THOUGHT HE WAS DREAMING when he saw two large breasts rise out of the misty hot tub, nipples shining like mountaintops awakening to another day. The woman, at one with nature except for a towel wrapped around her head, slowly walked up the steps from the tub, faced the drunk and nearly drunk party-goers enjoying the chilly April air and, after struggling to find the belt to her robe, very deliberately put it on. A redhead, with smaller breasts but long luscious legs, pulled herself out of the tub, walked over to the outside bar, refilled her glass of wine and handed it to a male companion. She stood for a moment, stretching her arms, then bending over to touch her toes before rejoining the merry-makers in the steam.

"Sammy . . . uh, Rachel . . . so glad you're here," yelled Sylvia Gordon, placing her wine glass on a small table twenty feet away and approaching them with the theatrical air of Tallulah Bankhead. "I just can't believe it's taken so long for us to get you over here, and you didn't even come in the front of the house?"

Sylvia was a tall, thin woman in her early forties with short-cropped, jet-black hair and a puckered face that looked like she'd just bitten into a Lemon Head. Her gold sequined dress dropped in the middle to reveal a generous amount of flesh and rose above her knees enough to confirm nice calves and hint at firm thighs. She gave each of them a from-the-bellybutton-up hug, making sure her lower body was well away from them, then banged on the sliding glass door separating the patio from the sunroom.

"Mo, look who's here," she yelled in a manner that would make a dock worker proud. "It's Sammy and his wife, uh . . ."

Sylvia looked at Rachel sheepishly, and Rachel responded with a fake grin, "Rachel. My name is Rachel."

Sylvia stopped her banging and looked at Rachel for a moment, then said, "Whatever."

Mo sauntered through the sunroom door and opened his arms. He was about five-nine, a good inch shorter than Sylvia, with perfectly coifed, curly hair. He had on a dark, tailored Italian suit with a loud tie that looked like it had been designed by someone on LSD. As he shook Sammy's hand and embraced Rachel, the diamonds on his watch shone like a star, matched in brilliance only by the emeralds on his cufflinks.

"Wow, what a home," Sammy said, his head moving to scan the stucco contemporary masterpiece.

Mo grabbed the two of them by the arms and led them toward the house. "You ain't seen nothing yet, Sammy, my boy."

"I'll be there in just a sec." Sylvia said and picked up her glass. "Gotta get a refill."

Mo, Rachel, and Sammy walked from the sunroom into the great room, which had a two-story, stacked stone fireplace as its centerpiece. The back of the house was glass and overlooked the Chattahoochee River. Mo led them to the right of the main room and on to a one-step landing in front of his dark-paneled study, where a fire burned in the pink marble fireplace.

"Everyone!" Mo yelled above the din. "I want you to meet my associate, Sammy Lansky, and his wife, Rachel." A few people clapped, some waved hello, but most of them just acknowledged Mo's interruption and continued their conversations. Sammy noticed that a few of the men had trouble taking their eyes off of Rachel. Though she wore relatively conservative clothes and little makeup, she still turned heads.

"Let's get you a drink and something to eat," said Mo, putting his arms inside those of Sammy and Rachel.

After a few more introductions, Mo guided them to the bar and the dining room. Sammy made small talk with some of the other doctors while Rachel hung around in silence, looking at her watch every fifteen minutes or so.

"There're big bucks galore here, huh, Rach?" he said as he stuffed a petite roast beef sandwich into his mouth.

Rachel reached for a napkin and used it to wipe mustard from Sammy's chin. "You better practice eating in public before you become rich." She looked for a place to put the napkin. "Anyway, I've had about as much of this fun as I can stand. Go talk to your buddies about the money, then let's split."

"Go?" Sammy said in a loud voice. "We just got here." He opened his arms toward the table of food. "I mean, look at all these fancy eats."

Rachel shook her head. "Give me a break, Sammy. To you, fancy means it comes in a can with an Italian label."

She stepped over to a nearby hunt board where she had placed her purse. "C'mon, James Beard, do your fact finding, then let's go." Rachel grabbed the purse, and at the same time Mo's meaty hand latched on to Sammy.

He whispered in Sammy's ear, "Me, Dellwood, and Henry would like for you to join us for a little private celebration, if you will, in the cabana."

Rachel looked at Sammy, then tried to step around Mo to extricate Sammy, but Sylvia grabbed Rachel first.

"Sweetie, come with me. I want you to meet some members of the medical auxiliary." They walked a few steps into the great room, Rachel firmly in Sylvia's clutches, and Sylvia continued.

"Did I ever tell you how happy Mo and I are to have Sammy as part of the team?" She spoke while looking around the room, never once turning to face Rachel. "Mo says Sammy is top notch. They're exactly the words he used: 'top notch.' We should've had you kids out here sooner. You know, Sammy has been with Mo now, what? . . ."

"Almost four years," Rachel deadpanned.

Sylvia turned toward Rachel for a second, then continued observing the other guests. "Well, with all my activities, who has time?"

Sylvia moved Rachel into the sunroom and sat her on a heavy, mint-colored sofa. "Did you know I'm membership chair this year at the club? God, what a job. Everybody wants to join. But we can't let just anyone join. After all, the club would loose its aurora—or is it aura?" This time Sylvia looked at Rachel when she spoke, but her dark eyes still darted around the room, keeping a close watch on everything.

"Well, anyway, I wish they had never insisted I take the job." Sylvia rose and kissed a tall, thin man who presented himself at her side. She sat again and said, "You know, we might have more in common than you think. I mean, you are rural and we are big city people, but being doctors' wives is our bond, don't you think? I'm sure we will become the best of friends over the years."

Sylvia rose and embraced a sleek woman wearing a dress that was open from her ankles to the top of her thigh. "Hello, Hilde, darling," Sylvia said.

"Your artwork, it's magnificent," Hilde said with an affect surely rehearsed in front of a mirror for hours. "Who is your art consultant?"

Sylvia waved her off. "Raoul Teffoia, but to call him an art consultant is stretching it. I mean, I had to practically whip the poor man to make him understand that people of means expect a certain level of service."

Hilde nodded and left. Rachel shook her head and watched as Sylvia ran off to kiss one of her guests. She sat for a moment, waiting for Sylvia to clear the room, then wandered into the dining room to wait for Sammy, who had disappeared with Mo.

Mo led Sammy into a glass conservatory that adjoined the great room, then outside by the pool, and into the large, detached cabana. He opened a beautiful set of French doors. Dellwood Dole and Henry Morton were sitting inside, perched on overstuffed chairs covered in Haitian cotton. The pink marble flooring reflected flames from the large stone fireplace. The room was not large, but it was completely filled with paintings and objets d'art.

Dellwood, dressed in an elegant black suit with a white silk shirt opened to the nipple line to reveal a gold necklace, rose and took Sammy's hand in both of his. "So good to see you, Sam, my boy," he said, rubbing Sammy's hand with his. "Yes, so good to see you on such a happy occasion: you becoming a millionaire." Sammy hated the shortened version of his name and he was sure Dellwood knew that.

Henry, dressed like a banker, also offered his moist, limp hand to Sammy. He was tall and thin with a narrow face that sported a beard and almost transparent skin. To Sammy, his head looked like a shriveled coconut with facial hair. Henry wore black, horn-rim glasses, and when he spoke, which was not often, his mouth moved so little that he looked like a bird.

"Nice to see you," he chirped. "I hope you are keeping well."

Sammy nodded.

"Whatcha have to drink?" Mo asked from the bar across the room.

Sammy shrugged. "Whatever you've got."

"What?" Mo yelled with a big smile on his face. "Come over here," he said, motioning for Sammy to join him at the bar. Sammy did as commanded, and when he got to the bar, Mo slapped him on the back. "You see this bar?" he asked, pointing to the large piece of dark wood. "This is no ordinary bar. You know why?"

Sammy shook his head.

Mo laughed again, put his arm on Sammy's shoulder, and said, "This bar came from The End of the World Pub in Kinsale, County Cork, Ireland."

"Wow," Sammy said softly.

"Yep," Mo continued. "My art man had it imported here just for me. But," he said, waving his index finger at Sammy, "that's not why it's special, son. Nope, it's special because it's a rich man's bar, and rich men don't drink 'whatever you got.'" He laughed again, then went behind the bar. "Rich men," he yelled, "drink this and this." He placed a bottle of twenty-five-year-old single malt MacCallan and a bottle of Dom Perignon on the bar, then laughed so hard he almost choked. When he had regained his composure, he said, "*Now* what would you like, Sammy?"

"The scotch, I . . . "

Sammy was interrupted by the bellowing of Dellwood's voice behind him. "Rosvita, darling, you look so divine."

Sammy turned around and saw Dellwood kissing the hand of a goddess who had entered the cabana while he was learning what rich men drink. She was a few inches taller than Dellwood, and had a carved face that virtually radiated light. She wore a plain, short, black dress, and she wore it elegantly. As soon as Sammy turned around and looked at her, she stared at him and smiled. Dellwood, looking from her face to Sammy's, took the woman by the hand and led her over to the bar.

"Sam, please meet the pride and joy of Munich, Fräulein Rosvita Schuler." Dellwood took the woman's hand and extended it toward Sammy, who hesitated for a moment, then shook it.

"Nice to meet you," he said in a quiet voice.

Sammy had known many women, even in the biblical sense, and many of them had been beautiful, but this Rosvita made him weak in the knees and gave him the cotton mouth like a six pack of Pabst Blue Ribbon.

Rosvita took Sammy's hand in both of hers and smiled at him. Her eyes were such a deep blue they were like natural pools. "I have heard a great deal about you, Dr. Lansky, and now I am pleased to meet you."

Sammy, trying to keep from staring at her, looked back at the bar, but when he turned back toward her, her high beams pointed right at him. For a few seconds, she stared, and he tried to avoid her eyes.

Dellwood relieved the tension by asking Rosvita if she wanted a drink.

"Champagne would be lovely," she answered.

Mo poured the champagne while Dellwood escorted Sammy and Rosvita to one of the couches where he placed the two of them side by side, then sat on an ottoman at their feet.

"Rosvita," Dellwood began as he crossed his legs, moved forward on his stool, and placed his hands on her knee, "has been *invaluable* in helping us with our current machine *and* in helping us plan for the future. Isn't that right, dear?" He ran his hand up her leg and squeezed her thigh.

She nodded and smiled without opening her mouth.

Dellwood took a sip of his drink, rose and walked over to the mantle, placing his glass on it. He leaned against the mantle, and the light from the fire reflected off his thick, gold necklace. "You see,

Sam, the delectable Rosvita is the vice-president for sales and marketing of the very company that manufactures the lithotriptor, Dornier Medical, North America, which just happens to be based right here in good old Atlanta. She and her company are very pleased with the work we have done through LithoServices, and—" He took another sip then resumed, "are looking forward to a wonderful future with us. Isn't that right, darling?"

She leaned forward, putting her drink on a small glass table. "Your machine," she said in accented English, "is now the busiest one in the whole of the country." She looked at Dellwood and Sammy as she spoke. "I think I can speak for the company when I say that we are proud and happy to be associated with you."

"Bravo," Dellwood bellowed, opening his arms as if to fly. He turned to Henry, who was standing next to Mo at the bar. "Henry, refill my glass while I kiss the hand of our guest." Dellwood returned to Rosvita and bent down to kiss her hand, but she shrugged him off. He stroked the back of her neck.

Henry brought the drink to Dellwood, who returned to his position by the fire. "We have done such a marvelous job in Georgia that we see no reason to, shall we say, sequester our talents." He took a large sip of alcohol and looked at Henry and Mo, both standing by the bar. "Therefore," he announced as he swept his blond mane back with his right hand, "we are going to take our management skills to all the other states with this kidney stone problem—Florida, North Carolina, Tennessee, South Carolina, Virginia, etcetera—offering the urologists there the same level of service we have given the doctors in this state."

Across the room, Mo raised his glass. "Cheers!" he saluted. "Here's to our success."

The private party ended when Dellwood finished his drink and headed for the door. As they walked out into the night, Rosvita tapped Sammy on the shoulder, and when he turned, she lightly stroked his arm then handed him a business card. He accepted it with a half-smile then, without saying anything, followed the others into the conservatory where some people were gathered around the piano singing Gene Pitney's "Only Love Can Break a Heart," and others were dancing.

Rachel spotted Sammy and grabbed him as soon as he was within arm's length. "It's time to go," she whispered in his ear and pinched his lower arm.

"But, Rach . . ."

Rachel spoke loudly to Sylvia, who was a few feet away. "Sylvia, we've got a long way to drive, so we better get going." Rachel looked up at Sammy, who forced a smile.

Sylvia waved but said nothing as she walked toward the hot tub. They found Mo, said goodbye, and left.

Still flushed from the premium scotch, the company of a beautiful woman, and the enormous success of his business venture, Sammy glowed. "Jesus, what a party," he said as they walked out through the front door. When they reached the valet parking desk the Gordons had set up for the evening, he asked his wife, "Have a good time?"

Rachel was silent.

"Looks like you two hit it off pretty well." When his enthusiasm was met with Rachel's blank stare into space, he clarified, "You and Sylvia, that is."

"I know whom you meant," Rachel answered without looking at him.

Sammy took some bills out of his pocket and handed them to the valet.

"I hate that woman," Rachel said with her jaw clenched.

"Huh? Why? What happened?" Sammy asked as he looked down the street for his car.

"She's everything I despise. She's selfish and self-promoting. There isn't one nice bone in her whole body." Rachel stared at him. "Need any other reasons?"

Sammy continued to look away from her. "Hey, I kind of thought you guys were getting . . ."

"You know what she told me? She and Mo don't like to socialize with the doctors from the south side of Atlanta because they're too low-class. The Gordons fancy themselves too sophisticated, too worldly. She went on and on about how wonderful she is, name-dropping at every chance. She spends more at the hairdresser than a lot of people in Atlanta make in a year. On and on." She grabbed Sammy by the arm, forcing him to look at her. "But you know what irked me the most? Not once in this whole 'I love me' fest did she mention her kids. Not once."

"She is kind of self-centered," Sammy said with a chuckle. "Acts like she's from money. Must be."

"Bullshit! One of her big buddies told me she's strictly Flatbush Avenue, Brooklyn; didn't have crap till Mo went into practice. Now she's looking down her long, should've-had-plastic-surgery-but-Daddy-couldn't-afford-it nose at everyone. Her friend told me you should consider yourself lucky if Sylvia will even speak to you. Well, I got news for Mrs. Morris Gordon. She doesn't have to worry about talking to me. If I *never* speak to her again, it'll be too soon." Rachel stepped out of her high heels and stood in the grass in her stocking feet.

"Ah, c'mon, Rach," Sammy said, putting his arm around her. "Usually people who act like that have an inferiority complex. I'll bet that's her real problem."

Their car arrived, they got in, and Sammy drove slowly away.

Rachel looked in the passenger vanity mirror, pulled her hair back and fashioned it into a ponytail. "Sammy, you're so blind sometimes it amazes me. After you went wherever with Mo, Sylvia took me around for about five minutes, then unceremoniously dumped me. I wandered into the kitchen to use the bathroom, and when I came out I overheard her telling one of her buddies that you reminded her of Jethro on *The Beverly Hillbillies*."

She turned to face him. "She said something like, 'He's so handsome. Tall, must be six-two or three, with dirty blond hair and green eyes. But when he opens his mouth, there goes the romance.' The bitch said I dress like I buy my clothes at the Junkman's Daughter, and the way I talk, my name ought to be Tammy or Wynonna. She told her big buddy Hilde that she didn't take me to the club because some of the members might think she had brought her domestic."

Sammy turned toward Rachel. "Shit, she said that?"

Rachel nodded. "Do you think she'd like your buddies from Cordele, like Clete or Stewball? Even worse, Big Boy Bates? How you think she'd feel coming to a party at your apartment with them?"

He thumped the steering wheel. "Ooh, be a damn disaster."

"Yet you like those guys. In fact, you love them. And not just because you grew up with them. They're your buddies because they're such good human beings. You'd do almost anything for one another." Rachel looked straight ahead. "She'd never give them a chance; they aren't her *kind of* people."

"Look, we've established that Mo and Sylvia, particularly Sylvia, aren't your type," Sammy said, raising his voice and peering at Rachel. "Let's drop it."

Sammy drove out onto I-285 and headed toward town.

"They've got too much. That's another thing that bothers me," she said, folding her arms.

"Hell, it doesn't bother me." He rolled down his window. "I'd love to get my share."

"Come on, Sammy. Think about the urologists in Ann Arbor we knew. Not just the ones at the university, but also the ones in private practice—Cal McHugh, Bobby Solomon, Carl Fisher. All of them were as busy as Mo, but none of them seemed to have his kind of money."

"Mo's a better businessman. I like that about him."

Rachel shook her head and sat sideways in the passenger seat. She pulled her legs under her and rubbed the bottom of her feet. "Oh, my God. What the hell have you gotten into? I mean, how did a guy with your training and your intelligence end up with a pair of low-lifes like the Gordons? This whole thing—business men with M.D. degrees, nude couples in hot tubs, people who think their shit doesn't smell—where the hell did you go wrong?"

She reached across the seat and rubbed Sammy's arm. He stared straight ahead. "You should leave, Sammy. Call one of the guys you trained under in Ann Arbor and see if they've got a job available. Call one of the guys down in South Georgia, Albany, or Americus; maybe they need someone. At least you'd be near your parents," she added.

Sammy stared straight ahead, his jaw clenched. "Ann Arbor's nowhere, Rachel, and those black holes south of here are less than nowhere. Atlanta's where it's happening." He looked at her. "I like the idea of making big bucks. You've got to be a businessman these days in medicine. You know I'm not one of those doctors who looks at patients and sees dollar signs. I just happen to like the idea of making money. Hell, ain't nothing wrong with having a little extra, is there?" He stopped talking and waited for her response.

Rachel turned on the radio, which was the only sound for the next several minutes as Sammy negotiated their way home. As they entered the driveway leading to the apartment, Rachel reached down to turn off the radio. "By the way," she said in a firm but quiet voice, "what did Mo say about the two checks?"

Sammy parked the car and opened his door. "Nothing much," he said as he stepped out. "Everything's okay, just as I thought."

Rachel opened her door and followed him into the apartment. As soon as they entered, she grabbed him by the back of his coat. "That answer," she said, shaking her head, "is a non-answer."

Sammy turned to face her, moving her hand off his coat as he did. "That's what he said, damn it."

She stared at him. He waved her off and began to climb the steps.

Rachel spoke in a clearly determined voice. "Tell me what Mo said before you take another step."

He turned around three steps up and said, "Nothing . . . he said nothing." Sammy then came down the steps and got right in Rachel's face. "That's not exactly true, Rachel." He was talking loudly now. "Mo did tell me two things: number one was that I needed to learn how rich folks live because, number two, they have plans for me to become really rich. And you know what?" He opened his arms as if preaching. "I think I'm gonna love it."

"Open your eyes, Sammy. These guys are no good; they aren't your real friends. Clete, Stewball, Big Boy—they're your friends." She took his hand and squeezed it. "Those other guys are losers," she said loudly. "And as long as you're with them, you're one, too."

Sammy threw her hand away and smiled. "What a joke, you calling *me* a loser—what a joke." He started back up the stairs as she yelled after him, and he didn't turn around.

"You, Sammy Lansky, are like a rainbow missing a few colors. You know what you call a rainbow like that?"

By now he had reached the top stair, where he stopped but still refused to turn and face her.

Rachel pretended to laugh. "Nothing, nada, zilch, a few insignificant colors in the sky."

He turned around and had the look of a madman on his face. "What makes you such a fucking expert on life? If you love my friends so much, why don't you go *marry* one of them?" With that, he turned the corner into the kitchen and out of sight.

Rachel was shaking badly now and could feel her heart pounding into her neck. Without saying another word, she marched upstairs, past Sammy who was rummaging in the refrigerator, and into the bedroom. A few minutes later, she emerged with a suitcase. Sammy was sitting at the dinette eating a sandwich.

"What the hell's that?" he asked with his mouth full.

Rachel started to speak, but her voice was very shaky, so she stopped for a second and tried to regain her composure. She began to cry, so without saying a word, she walked down the stairs slowly.

Sammy stood, wiped his lips, and finished the bite in his mouth. "Wait . . . wait a minute. What . . . what're you doing?" He pushed the dinette back and followed after her.

Rachel opened the front door, took a step outside, then looked back at him.

"Sammy." She had stopped crying, but her voice still quivered. "Have you ever thought about why we've stayed in this little apartment? I mean, we rented this place when we first got here with three pieces of furniture and two suitcases. God knows, we could afford better now."

"Shit, I'm the one who wanted to move," he said, his tone now less forceful.

She shook her head and smiled slightly. "You always said that, but whenever I'd line up a real estate agent, you were too busy."

He held the door and took a step toward her. Again he was filled with rage. "I'm a goddamn surgeon. I've got a real job—I'm lucky if I have time to take a crap. You're a teacher—you work from eight to three and have the summers off. Shit, you've got enough free time to move every year if you wanted."

"There you are," she said, dropping her suitcase and throwing her hands in the air. "The world according to Sammy Lansky. Thirty-nine years old, and he still thinks the sun revolves around him." She shook her head, and a closed-mouth smile filled her face.

"You know what you really need? You need a house with one door, fifty mirrors and no windows. You wanna know why? That way," she said, leaning against the door, "you can go in and look at yourself all the time without ever having to look at the outside world."

He started to interrupt her, but she wasn't finished. "You love this place because everywhere you look you can see your wonderful self. This ridiculous hall of mirrors," she told him, opening her arms in a panoramic fashion, "is perfect for you."

She tried to slam the door closed, but he held it open. "Goddamn it! That's enough. You act like you're some kind of big bargain. Shit! Living with you is like life without parole."

She paused then walked toward him and got close enough so he could feel her breath. "You can come back into my life when you find those missing colors. For now," she said while backing up a step and grabbing the doorknob, "I'm gone." As soon as she had spoken the last word, she slammed the door in his face.

CHAPTER FOUR

Rachel didn't run away from Sammy; she left him, the difference being she intended the whole thing to be temporary. So, the next day she called to say she was staying only a few miles away with Joan Moscowitz, whom they had both known as kids. Joan had been known as "Motor Mouth" Moscowitz in her younger days and, even with the small amount of contact Sammy'd had with her in recent years, he still felt the moniker fit. Since Rachel had arrived there late Saturday night, he was sure every Jew south of Macon who had a telephone knew about the breakup by lunch on Sunday. He only hoped that, just as the Angel of Death had passed over the Hebrew homes in Egypt, this bit of bad news missed his parents' home, at least until the following Friday when he was going to visit them for the weekend.

After he returned home from work on Monday, Sammy lay on his bed for several moments, then rolled over and looked at a photo of Rachel and him standing atop a sand dune at Sleeping Bear Dunes National Park in northern Michigan. It had been taken one rare weekend during his internship when he'd had more than one day off. He stared at the picture in the neat silver frame and remembered how much in love they'd been.

On Saturday afternoons, after working thirty-six consecutive hours without sleep, Sammy would arrive at their apartment in Ann Arbor. He'd look as if he'd been lost in the woods for a week. Rachel would bathe him in Dead Sea salts, shave him, feed him, and by five that afternoon they would be in bed with a bottle of wine. They would make love with such passion that they would fall asleep in each other's arms until the next morning at six, when he was gone again.

Sammy took a deep breath and wiped a tear from his eyes. She had always been so sexy and especially reckless in the beginning. They had met as kids at the synagogue in Fitzgerald, and met again years later at a party in Atlanta. They'd dated a few times but only platonically. Sammy smiled, getting an erection when he thought about that *first* night . . .

They returned to her apartment after a movie and, for the first time, she asked him in. He sat in the den while she went to her bedroom for something. Suddenly, the lights in the den were off, and the only light that remained was a very dim one in the kitchen. Rachel's image appeared out of the near dark.

"Have some wine?" she asked. "I've got a glass here for you."

"Sure."

He reached for the glass, but got a firm, erect nipple in his mouth instead. Rachel, still standing in front of him, took his hand and moved it down then back up her nude torso. She stopped, rubbing his hand on both nipples. After several seconds, she moved his hand further down her gently gyrating body. She was quite wet already, but the touch of his hand made her ooze. She moaned softly as she manipulated herself with his fingers, then kissed his hand. Rachel unzipped Sammy's pants and pulled them off by the legs. She sat astride him and began to kiss him furiously. Her lips were soft and sweet, and her tongue gently massaged the inside of his mouth. She removed her tongue, stood up on the sofa and massaged her warm, moist clitoris on his face. Moaning loudly, she slithered down his body, and started to kiss his face, his neck, his chest. Then she licked the head of his large, full penis, moving all around its circumference. She took it in, full-mouthed, and sucked on it gently. Sammy was on his way to another world when she mounted him, and the motion of her pelvis transported both of them to ecstasy. Without a word, they fell asleep in each other's arms.

Back in the present, Sammy sat up and used his sleeve to wipe the stream of tears, which now dripped down his cheeks. *If only Rachel understood me*, he thought. He rocked back and forth on the side of the bed, thinking about how he would explain her departure to Mama and Papa.

❖ ❖ ❖

FRIDAY, HE ARRIVED IN CORDELE ABOUT HALF AN HOUR BEFORE SUNSET and the beginning of Shabbat, the Jewish Sabbath. He had hoped to catch his parents at the store, but he knew it was too late, as they always left early on Friday so they could get home and begin preparations before sundown. He drove straight home, and when he pulled into the gravel driveway, he saw his parents waiting for him in front of their small, red brick rancher. This had been part of the ritual since 1964, Sammy's first year in college. His parents, their small stature and short, curly, gray hair making them look almost like siblings, rushed to him, and they hugged and kissed. Frieda looked around her son to his car.

"So," she said, still staring at his empty car, "this meshugass with you and Rachel is for real, no?"

Sammy opened his trunk and removed a small bag. *So Motor Mouth has struck again.* "I guess you heard that from Joan?" he asked softly as he closed his trunk. "Mama, this craziness, as you call it, is only temporary . . . I think."

Nathan stood by the side of the car and shook his head. "This Moscowitz girl, I know she is the daughter of a very fine man, but . . . sometimes I think she, maybe . . ." He hesitated for a moment to look at Frieda. "Just maybe she might *zich einreden a krenk.*"

Frieda shot him a look. "If she gets sick from talking too much, this is her trouble. Right now, we got our own meshugass. Come." She motioned for Sammy and Nathan to go inside.

Sammy took his bag, threw it over his shoulder by the strap, and put his arms around both parents, each of them more than a foot shorter than he. They walked toward the house.

"Well," Frieda said, taking one last look at the car, "if you want my opinion, she is separated from you, not me. If she wants to come visit us here, she is welcome any time." They got to the front door, and she stopped. "If it just so happens that you are coming, too, then maybe you give her a ride—keep you from being so lonely on the trip down here, no?"

Sammy's father threw his hands in the air. "Oiy, gevald!"

A smile stole across Sammy's face. He shook his head, and they walked into the little house. Nothing had changed in the twenty-two years since he had gone to college—the linoleum on the kitchen floor was spotless, the breakfast nook had two places set, and the small, paneled den with its rows and rows of books and pictures was still dark. But Sammy didn't need his eyes to know he was home, it was Friday night, and the weather had turned warm. He could smell the chicken, challah bread, and sweet, fruity tzimmes casserole, which meant Sabbath had arrived, and he could hear the constant whir of the attic fan. He had asked, even begged, his parents to get air conditioning. The answer was always the same: "In the old country, we didn't even have fans. These will do just fine, thank you."

They sat on tattered furniture in the den. There were no overhead lights, just small, unattractive lamps by the side of

Nathan's and Frieda's favorite chairs. On the cherry coffee table was a pitcher of homemade lemonade and two glasses filled with hot, tannic tea which looked like it came from the Everglades and which his parents referred to as *glezel tai*. In each glass was a spoon. A small plate with cubes of sugar lay by the glasses. From the way Frieda stared at the pitcher of lemonade as she poured him a glass, Sammy knew his mother's inquisitive mind had not moved off the subject of her daughter-in-law.

"So," she began. "When will this—what you call it?—temporary problem be resolved?"

Sammy took a sip. "Don't know."

His mother sat back and crossed her hands. "Why you don't know? The way I look at it, when you got a problem, you got a solution. All you got to do is look for it, no?"

Frieda glanced at Nathan as she stirred her tea. She put a cube of sugar between her front teeth, then put the glass to her mouth without removing the spoon, and drank the tea through the cube. Sammy had only seen the Lanskys and Rachel's parents, the Dziewinskis, drink tea this way. Frieda was small, no more than ninety pounds, and her soft, thin skin and rounded face gave her an angelic look, but when she focused her brown eyes on someone, she immediately got their attention. She looked up at Sammy, shook her head, and spoke.

"None of this would have happened if you had roots in your marriage," she said.

Sammy stirred in his chair and thumped the side of his glass. He knew what was coming next, so he girded himself.

"Every time a Jewish child is born," his mother instructed as she had many times before, "the Nazis, they die again. You and Rachel have a child, then you wouldn't have time to worry about whatever got you in this mess."

Sammy sighed audibly. "Mama, we've been through this. We've tried, and it just hasn't happened."

Frieda put down her glass and wagged her finger at Sammy. "Well, I'm no doctor, but I know for sure that with you living alone and Rachel living with Joan—this way it will never happen."

Nathan saw the beads of sweat forming on his son's face. "Schmuel," he said, using his son's Hebrew name and offering him the plate. "Have some mandel bread. Mama just made it."

"Not too much!" Frieda pulled the plate away from Sammy after he'd taken one piece of the crumbly treat. "I made a big dinner for tonight."

"You," Frieda said, again waving a finger at Sammy, "are too hard to please. You have a wonderful girl, good where it counts." She raised her voice when she said the last word and pointed to her heart. "And you don't have enough sense to keep her happy. *This* is what I call the craziness."

Sammy looked heavenward. "Oh, God, please."

"I think," Nathan interrupted, "that Rachel's parents poisoned her." He paused for a second, looking first at Sammy, then Frieda. "Maybe that's why she and Schmuel, they have this problem, Mama."

Frieda waved him off. "What do Avrum and Ester Dziewinski have to do with Rachel and Sammy having a baby? I ask you this and also tell you that talking of the dead in such a way—this is not done—certainly not on Shabbat." She placed her glass on the table with a thump. "Plus, the past, it is the past." She paused and looked at Sammy. "What matters is today and tomorrow."

Sammy shook his head in frustration. "We split because . . . "

"Mama and I have done everything we can so that our lives, our thoughts, our spirits would move out of Europe," Nathan said, ignoring his son. "This has been very hard. Mind you, we do not want to forget the past, but to live in it is wrong. Your mother and I . . ." He turned to Frieda, and their eyes met. "We made a pact when we married that our lives would not be a memorial to our dead, but would bring to them much honor. You understand?"

"Sure," Sammy replied. "But, that didn't have anything . . . "

"Avrum Dziewinski," Nathan continued, "he did not do this. He lost two children in Europe, but he had another beautiful one after he came to this country. He was so afraid of losing her, he made her miserable."

"Nathan." Frieda raised her index finger in the air. "You are overstepping your bounds."

"It's okay," Sammy said. "Rachel's told me the same thing. But when she got away from them, she was fine, just like I told you. Let's change—"

"I think Avrum killed whatever spirit his wife Ester had left after the Nazis got through with her," Nathan continued. Sammy sighed, knowing full well that his father had a way of getting his agenda across despite any opposition.

"She was almost a prisoner in her own house. When he died, Ester didn't know how not to be a prisoner—first the Germans, then Avrum. They, both of them, let the Nazis destroy their souls." Nathan pounded his fist against the table. "I would as soon have died in Auschwitz as to let them do that to me."

Sammy abruptly clapped his hands. "Enough! Rachel escaped from her parents. Don't try to put her back in prison, as you call it."

Nathan stirred his tea. "I say one more thing—to get it off my shoulders—then I shut up."

"Praise God," Frieda said, rising to check the dinner.

Nathan took a sip, placed his glass on the table, and spoke. "I tell you, I know about Avrum and Ester's past, and if they thought this was so great, so wonderful that they wanted to live in it, they must have been more meshuggenah than I thought."

"Nachum!" Frieda yelled from the kitchen, addressing her husband by his Hebrew name. "Enough! *Es past nit!* We eat now. We no longer talk about these things."

Nathan put his hands in the air and stood. "Okay. *Genug ist genug.* I say no more."

Sammy, still sitting, shook his head as he rose and followed his parents into the light gray dining room off the kitchen.

Frieda covered her head with a napkin and waved her hands over two lit candles while chanting a prayer, thereby ushering in the Sabbath. Nathan said the blessings over the bread and wine. They ate in silence for several moments. Frieda watched as Sammy filled his plate with chicken, tzimmes, noodle kugel, and kasha, then she shook her head and said, as she had for years,

"What, you're not hungry? You don't like the food? You get better cooking somewhere else? Maybe you stopped on the way home and ate that *traif* on the roadside, no?"

Sammy laughed and gave his usual answer. "I've got only one stomach. Do I look like a cow?"

"Let him eat in peace, Mama," Nathan said.

They ate. Sammy and Nathan told Frieda how wonderful the food was. After another brief period of silence, Sammy wiped his mouth and spoke. "You know, maybe the Dziewinskis lived too much in the past, but sometimes, I mean, I'd kind of like to know more about what y'all went through in Europe." He leaned back in his chair. "You know, not all the gory details, but what it was like, more about how we got here. I mean, we've talked about it and all, but y'all always want to change the subject when we really start getting to the nitty-gritty."

There was a moment of silence. Sammy, seated between the two, placed a hand on each of his parent's arms and spoke to fill the void and ease his discomfort. "I don't need to be protected anymore.

You guys have protected me from what went on in Europe so well it's kind of like my life didn't start until we moved to America, and I know full well that isn't so." He looked from parent to parent. "No one's coming to get us, take anything away from us, or hurt us in any way. The past *is* the past, but your past is also my past, and I deserve . . . I need to know more about it."

Frieda stopped eating, looked at Nathan, then spoke. "You know that Papa and I met after the liberation of Auschwitz and that we went to Treviso in Italy where you were born. From there to Cyprus and then to Atlanta, then here. What more is there to tell? Plus the fact that with our darling Rachel missing from the table, we've got more important matters to discuss."

Sammy put his arms on the table. "Well, I mean, what about your families? I've got aunts, uncles, cousins who I've never met and will never meet. What about them?" He looked back and forth from parent to parent. "It's time, Mama and Papa. None of us is getting any younger, so you need to tell me. I need to know everything about my . . . our past."

There was silence as Frieda got up, moved her chair back, and walked through a swinging door into the kitchen to get more food. She returned and offered some to Sammy and Nathan. Then, after putting the platter on the table, with the serving spoon still in her hand, she spoke.

"There is not much to tell, Sammy. I was born Fruma Prelesnik in a village east of Lodz, Poland. My family was taken by the Nazis and killed. I survived by working in the Lodz ghetto." She peered up at her husband. "I went to Auschwitz in 1944." As she looked heavenward, she recounted, "Thanks, God, the Russians, they came and liberated us."

"I know all of that," Sammy said.

"See," she said as she sat. "You know more than you think."

"C'mon, Mama."

She took a bite and said nothing. Sammy looked at his father. "Why didn't you and your family leave when you could?"

Nathan shrugged his shoulders and furrowed his brow. "No one believed the Nazis that they had plans to kill all the Jews. And, where would we go? No one wanted us." He shrugged, took a drink of water, shook his head.

After a pause, he continued, "For some reason, they—the officials in these countries like Poland and Russia—blamed us for everything they did wrong." He laughed softly. "We, the Jews who were not citizens, did not own land, weren't allowed to go to school. Why were we so important they had to worry about us?"

Several moments of silence followed. The only sound was that of food being eaten. Frieda began to tap her fingers on the table, then rose and walked into the kitchen. She brought in a marble cake and fruit. "Try the strawberries, Sammy. We just got them in today." She cut a large piece of the cake, put it on Sammy's dessert plate, then scooped some big, shiny strawberries on top. As she started around the table toward Nathan, he began to speak again.

"You know, Schmuel, the thing what always amazed me was that six million Jews died forty years ago, and one Jew died two thousand years ago. The one what died so long ago, they talk about him every day." He paused while Frieda put the cake and fruit on his plate. "The others—the six million—they get mentioned only once in a while." He stopped talking and shook his head.

Frieda bent down and kissed her husband. "Don't give him a philosophy course." She stood up and walked toward her seat. "Just eat the cake, eh, Papa?"

He put his small hands on top of his son's. Sammy could see the letter and four numbers tattooed on his father's forearm. "My family in Bialystok was arrested and killed, but I managed to escape and join the partisans."

"I remember you telling me that. Did you kill any Nazis?" Sammy asked. "I mean, as a partisan?"

Nathan didn't reply. Frieda took a bite of the cake, and as she spoke, Sammy noticed that her hand trembled. "Your father," she said, looking at Nathan, "lived as a partisan for a year and a half. In the winter of 1944, he and a few comrades made it to Budapest and got fully involved with the effort to save the Jews there by distributing false papers. He was caught trying to get someone out and was taken to Auschwitz."

Sammy looked at his small, peaceful father and smiled but said nothing.

Nathan removed his hands from Sammy's. "Well, you know the rest. Your mother and I met after the camp was liberated by the Red Army in . . . what month was that, Mama?"

"January, 1945." Without looking at her son, Frieda put the cake to her mouth, then put it down without taking a bite. "We met then, but we left the camp in February," she said in a soft voice that cracked as she spoke.

Sammy eyed his mother for a moment, then turned to his father. "Did you kill any SS?" he asked. "I read somewhere that the Russians let the prisoners do whatever they wanted to the SS."

Nathan shook his head. "There were three thousand people breathing and three million not breathing when the camp was liberated." Nathan spoke in monotone as if to divorce himself from the subject. "I say it this way because so many of those who had survived were *muselmen*, the living dead. Soon, they would join the others who had died. We hated the SS, but they were no longer our main concern."

"Damn, I would've hunted down the bastards as soon as I was strong enough." Sammy grabbed the cake knife in his hand and squeezed it. "You were a partisan, Papa. You could've handled those SOBs."

Frieda and Nathan glanced at each other. "We had had enough of killing," Frieda said, barely audible.

"Killing was too good for those bastards." Sammy said, using the knife to cut a piece of cake in one swoop. "They needed to be tortured."

"We had a chance once," Nathan said quietly, looking down at his hands and rubbing them together.

Sammy chewed the cake. "A chance to kill a Nazi?" he asked.

His father nodded. "Yes," he answered. He looked at Sammy with his hazel eyes narrowed, and after a moment, he began.

"The details are unimportant, son, but I did have the chance once. There he was cowering in front of me, helpless like so many of my people had stood in front of him. I had practiced what I would say if I ever got such an opportunity." Nathan raised his voice.

Frieda began to clear the table. "Enough of the dramatics. We stop talking about this now. No one is coming back to life because of this conversation."

Nathan handed her his plate and continued as if he hadn't heard her. "I wanted to kill him." He stared toward a corner of the room. "I wanted to yell at him, not to scare him, but to let him know that we were no longer the *untermensch*, the subhumans, that he thought we were." He turned toward Sammy and sighed. "I wanted to let him know that I was better than he was because I had survived the worst nightmare he could have devised. In a war of will, I had won."

Nathan was quiet for second. He puckered his lips and spoke, rubbing his son's hand as he did. "When I looked at this animal, I did not see a human being, but I could not kill him."

"Why?" Sammy asked, leaning over and placing his hand on his father's shoulder.

Nathan shook his head. As he began to speak, the swinging door opened and Frieda reentered. "There is an old Yiddish saying," he said as he kissed his son's hand. "In the times of war, the devil, he makes more room in hell. I had been to hell already. Killing this animal wouldn't change that."

"*Gottenyu,*" Frieda yelled. "That is a German proverb." She pointed her index finger at Nathan. "Nowhere in Yiddish do you find this type of heaven and hell thing. You are rambling on and doing nothing but stirring up the past." She made circles with her hands as she said this.

Nathan shot her a serious look. "Sammy asked me if I ever had a chance to kill a Nazi. I am giving him an answer."

"I want to hear no more stories like this tonight," Frieda insisted, turning to Sammy and throwing her hands in the air. "Your father gets carried away sometimes. We went to Treviso, where we were married and you were born. From there, we tried to enter Palestine but were interned on Cyprus. Thanks God, Mr. Erwin Rich in Atlanta and some other businessmen helped us get to Atlanta, then we came here to Cordele and have been here ever since. That's enough for tonight." She shot a look at her husband. "Stories about killing, they don't need to be told." She stared at Nathan for a moment, then looked sternly at Sammy.

"We have to get up early in the morning to go to shul. Maybe we say a prayer that Rachel, she and Sammy can get over their differences, no?" She stormed out of the dining room toward the bedroom.

Father and son sat in silence, listening to the attic fan. Sammy leaned over, hugged his father, and said, "I love you, Papa.

◆ ◆ ◆

THAT NIGHT, SAMMY TOSSED AND TURNED, TRYING TO SLEEP. He would have killed the Nazi and enjoyed every moment. About three o'clock in the morning, he heard noise from his parent's bedroom. Their door creaked open and he could hear his father whispering, "Calm down, Fruma. It's okay, my dear."

Sammy arose and saw his father holding onto his mother and taking her toward the kitchen. He slipped quietly into the hall and watched as Nathan sat her at the table, then put on a kettle to make tea. While the water was heating up, Nathan stood behind her rubbing her shoulders. She had her head resting on her arms, and Sammy could hear her weeping. All of a sudden, Frieda sat up and began to wail in Yiddish: *"Mare kinder nicht! Bitte, sorgt ihm. Mare kinder nicht, Nachum."* ("No more children! Please, tell him. No more children, Nachum.")

Nathan rubbed her shoulders and kissed her neck. "We are in America now, Fruma, there will be no more killing." She rocked back and forth, weeping the whole time. The kettle whistled, Nathan poured some tea and sat next to his wife. They drank in silence for a short period of time, and then he began to hum a haunting melody. Frieda put her tea down, nodded at him and hummed with him. In a matter of seconds, they put words to the music: *"Henai matov uma n'ayim shevat achim gam yachad."* ("How wonderful it will be to dwell with our brothers again.")

Sammy had seen this many, many times in the past, but he had no idea what the whole thing was about.

CHAPTER FIVE

NACHUM AND FRUMA MET IN AUSCHWITZ after being liberated by the Red Army in January of 1945. They were two of only three thousand pitiful souls alive or partially alive in the belly of that beast. After a month in which they regained a small amount of strength, the couple left Auschwitz on foot and headed west. They trod, step by step, through the desolate landscape that was Upper Silesia. The road was strewn with dead and dying survivors of Birkenau and Auschwitz. Their striped pashkas held together by lice, these "victorious" victims of the Final Solution moved en masse to nowhere. As they marched, the cold wind blew through their garments like one last slap. Mercifully, some fell, never to rise again. Finally, after years, they had peace.

◆ ◆ ◆

"FRUMA, WE MUST GET OFF THIS ROAD and find better shelter. These KA-Zed garments will let us freeze," said Nachum, pulling at the thin concentration camp uniform.

"Nachum, I can't . . . Ahhhhhhhh!"

Nachum turned around and jumped back. In front of him, just on the edge of the woods, stood an SS officer, who spoke to him in German.

"I will not harm you, Jew. I want only your clothes. The war is over. I must get back to my family and rescue them from these Russian beasts. They have crossed the River Oder and these Red vermin will be moving toward the fatherland soon. Surely you can understand what these animals will do to my people. I must get to my family."

Nachum said nothing.

"Look, Jew, I will not leave you naked. You will have my clothes. The Russians will know you are not one of us, and they will let you pass. Show them your tattoo."

Nachum rubbed his arm. The letter and four numbers had been his name for a year.

The officer looked around and saw a barely breathing corpse lying three meters from Nachum. "You are in luck, Jew. I have found a better fit for my disguise. Surely he will be a willing contributor to the salvation of the Master Race." He nudged the nearly dead man with his foot. The man rolled over, and his cadaverous face, like so many of the walking dead in the camps, looked at the Nazi without expression.

"Schwein Jude!" The SS man kicked the final breaths from him, grabbed the Jew's striped uniform, and disappeared into the forest.

Nathan lay down next to Frieda in the deep snow. The cold, wet, February wind whipped through the pines. The trees swayed back and forth like the prisoners he had seen at one roll call after another in Auschwitz-Birkenau.

That night, this nameless road in Upper Silesia was filled with an exotic caravan of those liberated from German camps. On makeshift sleds hastily nailed together, they dragged small trunks and bundles—their worldly possessions. People who had been human refuse a few days before marched aimlessly. There were Bosnians, Slovaks, Czechs, Poles, Hungarians, all flying national flags fabricated at the last minute from German bedding. Then there were the Jews. What flag would they carry?

At sunrise, Nathan stirred and pulled himself out of the snow. His feet, hands, and lips were numb. He felt Fruma's chest move and knew she had survived another night. The caravan had moved on, and the road was empty. The glare of the rising sun impaired Nachum's vision, but he thought he saw a train on the road heading west. He walked toward it, shielding his eyes with his hand, and as he got closer, he realized the "train" was a long line of military trucks.

A Red Army major, standing at the front of the convoy, spotted the striped, ragged person approaching. He rolled a *machorka* between his fingers, took a deep drag, climbed on the running board, and casually observed the vehicles under his charge. The massive trucks, loaded high, snaked beneath the branches of the trees along the roadside. Machine guns, their volleys like hail on empty tin pots, rapped at Messerschmidts overhead in the wintry sky. The major looked at Nachum and, in Russian, asked who he was.

Nachum was silent.

"*Jude?*" asked the major.

"Yah," replied Nachum.

"Where are you from?" asked the major.

"Auschwitz."

The Russian took another drag on his cigarette and laughed. "No one is from Auschwitz. You go to Auschwitz, but you are not *from* there. What is your name, Yiddisha?"

Nachum rubbed his left arm. "Nachum."

"Are you by yourself, Mr. Yiddisha? What did you say? Nachum? Nachum what?"

"Zychilinsky." Nachum pointed to the road where Fruma now sat resting against a tree.

"So, this is your wife?"

"No. She is my friend."

"Where are you going, Jew? Oh, excuse me, I should know the answer to that question. For centuries, you brave descendants of Abraham have prayed to go back to your homeland. Now, now, my Yid friend, there are so many problems, no one gives a shit about you or your brothers. Every year, the Jews in my village would pray, 'Next year in Jerusalem. Next year in Jerusalem.' Well, Hitler proved to be your messiah. Go to Palestine. No one gives a damn."

"I will go to Treviso," said Nachum.

"Italy. Ha! Why would a Jew go to Italy? You people are swine, but you are better than the Italians."

"I have friends in Italy." He hoped the major would leave it at that. Nachum had heard about Operation Bricha being organized in Northern Italy's Treviso. This was to be the conduit to get Jewish refugees out of Europe for good.

The major inhaled the last of his cigarette and shouted something to his men, which made them laugh. "Get in the truck, Yid. We will take you and your friend as far west as the Elbe. From there, you are on your own. But first—first, we are going to let you in on a little fun. Let's go pick up your friend." The major got in the cab, motioned for Nachum to grab on to the side, then they picked up Fruma.

The convoy went about ten kilometers. The major leaned out of the cab and yelled something in Russian. Several soldiers jumped from the truck and into other vehicles, which took off down the road. The convoy now gone, the lone truck turned past a stone fence, down a gravel path, into a clearing, stopping by a Russian armored vehicle parked in front of a small stone house.

"Now, let's go inside for a little fun," said the major, leading Nachum and Fruma into the building.

In the main room were five or six Russian soldiers, the red insignia of General Zuchov's troops emblazoned on their sleeves. They were passing around a bottle of vodka and laughing. The major spoke, pointing to the disheveled man and woman brought into his lair. "The revenge of the people of Abraham will begin now. Come. We have business in the next room."

The soldiers laughed and clapped in response. Nachum, Fruma, and the major walked down a dark, narrow hallway and into a small bedroom. On the bed was a nude woman, her buttocks pointing to the ceiling, leather straps about her knees and wrists fastened to the bedposts holding her in position across the bed. Soldiers were taking turns with her, grunting as they shoved themselves inside. The woman made no noise.

Nachum and Fruma had seen the SS have this kind of "fun" so many times it left them unfazed. They heard only the rhythmic sound of the pendulum clock above the bed.

"Here is our present to you," said the major.

He pointed to the closet and pushed the two of them in that direction. They stood face to face with an SS officer. A rope tied his hands and held him to a hook, suspending his body a foot above the floor. The Nazi was naked to the waist—his SS tattoo peering beneath his armpit, a yellow star pinned to his bare chest. On the floor by the Nazi's boots lay a striped KA-Zed jacket. Nachum looked into the soldier's face. This was the man he had seen the night before, the man who had killed the Jew; he now wore the dead Jew's star.

The major handed a pistol to Nachum and screamed, "Shoot him, Jew!"

Nachum was shaking so hard he had to hold the pistol with both hands. Unable to stop trembling, Nachum handed the pistol back to the Russian.

"Shoot him, Jew dog!" yelled the officer as he shoved the gun yet again into Nathan's chest, placing the man's quaking hands around the weapon.

Nachum had shot Germans and blown up their trains, but that had been anonymous and impersonal. He had prayed for the chance to tell a German, one individual German, what he thought of their so-called solution, and now he had his chance.

He looked at the SS insignia and wanted to scream, "You are the master race, determining who shall live and who shall die. I am the filthy, lice-infested Jew, the *untermensch*. Scream that you are human, for I will show that your blood is as red as the blood of my *mishpucha* you killed yesterday. Yell at me as you did, and I will pour you into the fire of your own crematorium. Brutalize me one last time, so that all of your crimes will be punished."

He held the trigger tightly, closed it slowly, but did not fire.

"Ach, Jew!" screamed the Russian, "We have been to Auschwitz, remember? We were the ones who liberated you. We saw the piles of ashes twenty meters high. How many of your family were in those ashes, huh, Jew? Kill him! Kill him! Avenge your brothers!"

The SS officer, his blue eyes popping out of their sockets like huge bubbles, urinated and vomited.

Nachum knew it was time for the Jews to fight back. Masada had been almost nineteen hundred years ago. He would fight back if he could get to Treviso.

The Russian spit at Nachum. "Well, Jew, I guess you are cattle after all." He grabbed the gun, put his giant paw on Nathan's throat, and threw the smaller man across the room into a wall. There was silence for a moment. All Nachum could hear was his breathing, the clock, and groans from the bed.

Suddenly, the major went to the woman, who still had a young Russian mounted on her. The soldier grunted and rolled aside as the major pulled the woman's hair so that her contorted face, with its bulging, frightened eyes looked up at him, then he placed the gun in her mouth and fired two shots. Blood splattered over the clock as the pendulum maintained its rhythm. The major signaled for the soldiers to continue their merriment.

"That was for Stalingrad."

The major returned to the Nazi officer, pulled down his pants, and shot him in the groin. The SS man screamed as his organ exploded and his testicles leapt across the room.

"This is for Leningrad." The major grabbed a large, curved knife from his belt, stabbed the man above the bellybutton and ripped the knife down to the pubis.

"Take this pig outside! Feed him to the wild animals. I'm sure they are hungry after a long winter."

The soldiers left the dead woman and began to carry out the orders. The major wiped his hands on the filthy, striped garments and led Nachum and Fruma into the front room, where the men were dancing and singing.

"It's time to go," the major yelled to his troops. "We will have more fun as we get closer to the front." He motioned for the men to follow him as he pushed the Jewish pair outside.

From the front of the little house, they could see the dust of the Red Army in the near distance. It was as if someone had opened the floodgates and a river of metal flowed forward to Berlin led by Slavs with Red Kolpaks. Nachum wondered how many homes of Upper Silesia had flown the Swastika last week and now flew the Polish freedom flag. How many Polish women, who last week had rolled in bed with their SS lovers, were now throwing their naked flesh into the arms of the Red Army?

Fruma and Nachum made it to Treviso and got close enough to Palestine to see snow on Mount Carmel. However, the merchant marine ship trying to smuggle them into Palestine never made it, and they ended up in a refugee camp on the island of Cyprus.

The Atlanta Jewish Federation had tried to get a number of Holocaust survivors out of Europe. They offered to support them temporarily, teach them English, help them get jobs, and, in general, ensure that these refugees would not be a burden to the American taxpayer. The quantity of bureaucratic red tape proved to be almost insurmountable, and the naked, terrible truth was that no government was opening its doors to these desolate people. Europe was in a state of upheaval, as many of the survivors moved from one Displaced Persons camp to another. The Jews were stateless.

Erwin Rich, a prominent Atlanta businessman, proposed a new idea. Why not offer passage to refugees in Displaced Persons camps on Cyprus, many of whom had been waiting to enter Palestine for over a year? The British, who had detained them there, would be happy to see them leave. By this time, the British merely wanted to get out of Palestine themselves. Anyone who could take a few Jews off their hands was welcome to do so. Plus, no one really knew if or when Partition was going to occur, so many of these poor detainees might languish on Cyprus for the near future.

Fruma and Nachum, now married and using the family name Zychilinsky, didn't want to leave Cyprus. They were so close to the Promised Land, and they knew God's hand would guide the nascent United Nations along the proper path. Arabs and Jews would each have a homeland—partition of Palestine would assure that. But the Zychilinskys also knew they had to leave. They had a baby now, Schmuel, named after Fruma's beloved uncle, and he had been sick since their arrival on Cyprus. The British army doctor had said something about parasites causing his crippling diarrhea. He was almost two years old, yet he weighed only twenty pounds, and his eyes and belly seemed to be sucked in by a vacuum. There was something more terrible and disturbing about the baby: They had never seen him smile.

On the ship bound for America, Nachum and Fruma decided they would sever their last ties with Europe—they became Nathan and Frieda Lansky, and they called their son Sammy.

◆ ◆ ◆

ERWIN RICH HAD A PROBLEM. The Jews who had been lucky enough to emigrate from Europe in the thirties assimilated relatively easily into American culture. Those who came over right after the war had many problems. They were malnourished, poor, and in desperate psychological condition. The condition of the immigrants who had languished in Displaced Persons camps for years, such as the Lanskys, was worse than Rich could have imagined.

The postwar economy in Atlanta was booming, but what would he do with these poor humans whom no one else wanted? There was a shortage of housing and, even when he found work for them, their wages put them barely over subsistence. Saul Tatel, a merchant in Fitzgerald, a small, southern Georgia town, had an answer for Rich's dilemma. The young Jews who had been reared in places like Fitzgerald, Tifton, Oscilla, Unadilla, and Cordele weren't coming back after they went to college. Soon, the lack of Jews would reach the crisis point, and eventually the community would die. Saul Tatel vowed not to let that happen. If he couldn't entice the young adults to return to their hometowns, he would have to import recently immigrated Jews to rural south Georgia.

With family in tow, Nathan Lansky moved to Fitzgerald and went to work for Saul Tatel. Eventually, after five or so years, the

Lanskys moved again, this time to a larger town west of Fitzgerald, where there was a store for sale. Lansky's Market, 496 Tenth Street, Cordele, Georgia, became well known. It was in an old, two-story building with wooden floors that creaked. A green and white awning sheltered the front windows from the southern Georgia sun. The store was old but clean and had fresh produce and grade-A meat. In the summer they sold slices of chilled melon from a tub of shaved ice, and there was always a metal soda box filled with RC Cola and Coca-Cola. Every year, during the various seasons, Frieda would artistically arrange a produce table with corn, peaches, tomatoes, or peanuts.

The Lanskys had a pretty good business, but they were always the immigrants, the odd ones who looked and talked differently. It was not until ten years after their arrival they knew they belonged in this south Georgia outpost.

It was December of 1957, and the Lanskys, along with the few other Jews in Cordele, were celebrating Chanukah, the festival of lights. Frieda placed a small menorah in the front window of their home, and each night during the holiday, the family would light candles in it. Others had much larger and more elaborate menorahs, but none had one that was as special as Frieda's, for she had gotten her little brass one from her father before he was taken. Because it was so small, she had been able to hide it from the guards in Auschwitz.

One night during Chanukah, someone broke the glass in the Lansky's front window and smashed the menorah. The next day, the mayor of Cordele, a deacon in the Baptist church, went to Atlanta and visited the Temple, the Ahavath Achim Synagogue and the Beth Jacob Synagogue. At each place, he bought all of the menorahs they had. That night, after he returned, there were menorahs burning brightly in homes all over Cordele.

The words written by Emma Lazarus for the Statue of Liberty rang true. There would be no more Hitlers, no more Czars, no more ghettos, no more pogroms—the Lanskys were finally free.

CHAPTER SIX

THE NEXT MORNING, SAMMY PACKED HIS PARENTS into the back seat of his Saab and headed toward the synagogue in Fitzgerald, forty-five minutes away. By mutual agreement, he raised the front seat headrests so it would be difficult for normal-sized individuals to see out the front window; Frieda and Nathan, therefore, could see only out the side, which suited them just fine. They didn't like the way their son drove, and he didn't appreciate their running commentary on it—what they couldn't see didn't bother them as much. Nothing was said about last night's discussion nor about his mother's recurring nightmare, and Sammy decided to let things go for now. He looked in the rearview mirror, saw his parents holding hands, and smiled. They had traveled a long way together.

"Nathan, you remember the first time we drove this road by ourselves? It was . . . what? Forty years ago, no?" Frieda asked as they headed down Highway 107, east toward Fitzgerald.

Sammy checked the mirror again. He could tell by the smile on his father's face that he was about to hear, for at least the one thousandth time, the story of how Nathan learned to drive. Sammy looked forward and braced himself. He had memorized the story, so as a game, he tried to follow along with his father, word by word.

"Of course, I remember, dear," Nathan started. "Mr. Tatel, *olov hasolem*, came to me one day and said, 'Nathan, I want you to start delivering groceries on one of my west routes. You can make a lot more money. You can drive, can't you?'

"'Yes, yes,' I said, lying since I had never driven an automobile." Sammy joined his father for the next line in the story: "'Thank you, Mr. Tatel.'"

"What is that you said, Sammy?" his father asked.

Sammy looked at the road. "Nothing, Papa. Just talking to myself."

"The next day, we left you, Sammy, with one of the other families living in the old synagogue, walked to the alley behind the building, and got into a loaded delivery truck. One of the other deliverymen, realizing that the truck in front of him had not moved for ten minutes, got out of his vehicle to see what was going on. There he sees your mother and me pulling on the choke, begging the truck to go into first gear." Frieda and Nathan laughed.

Nathan spoke while Frieda was still giggling. "This man says to me, 'Vos tut zich?'"

Frieda stopped laughing. "The man was Mr. Wallace, Nachum. He never knew a word of Yiddish in his whole life."

"You're right," Nathan said, raising his hands. "I used the Yiddish to make it more interesting. Anyway, he asks what we're doing, then teaches us to drive right then and there, and that was the first time we go on this road."

"You know, your father, he is learning." Frieda met Sammy's eyes in the rear view mirror. "It used to take him . . . what? Fifteen minutes to tell that story. Now," she teased, pinching Nathan's cheek as she poked fun at him, "only a few sentences, it takes him." She laughed.

"You know why I have had to force such a beautiful and funny story into a little one?" Nathan put two fingers close together when he said the word *little*. "Because," he said, wagging a finger at Frieda, "you are forever saying to me, 'Gib zich a shockel, gib zich a shockel,' get on with the story. So," he mock surrendered, shrugging his shoulders, "I am forced to deny my son the pleasure of such a great story."

They laughed, and when Sammy looked in his rearview mirror again, his mother had her head on Nathan's shoulder.

They drove the last fifteen minutes down Highway 107 in silence. Sammy looked at the flat landscape with its scrub pines and dilapidated houses. This was a run-down part of Georgia with everything up on blocks. A lot of people said the tar-paper houses had foundations of four quadrants of stacked concrete blocks to allow the air to circulate better during the prolonged summers. That was a good explanation and was better than saying poor people just couldn't afford a decent foundation. The cars, rusted and missing pieces here and there, sat on concrete while their tires adorned the front yard. With all the junk outside the houses, including old wringer washing machines, it was hard to tell whether the people lived inside or out.

Sammy had few fond memories of this journey down 107. After the Lanskys had moved to Cordele, the only reason to go to Fitzgerald was either to attend synagogue or something related to it, like religious school, or Bar Mitzvahs. He used to sit in the back of his parents' ancient Buick and promise himself once he left home, he'd never set foot in the Fitzgerald synagogue again. For the most part, he'd been successful, so he really couldn't complain. Yet the passing flat landscape conjured up memories Sammy wanted to bury.

As smart as he had been in regular school, Sammy could never get too interested in religion or religious school. It hadn't been just Judaism that made no sense to him. He had gone to the Baptist church with his buddies, and all the talk of burning in hell gave him the willies. What really had made no sense to Sammy was that supposedly the Baptists didn't drink, smoke or dance, yet the biggest hell-raisers he knew were Baptists—including Reverend H. G. Hollingsworth of the Holiness Baptist Church of Cordele. Rumor had it that since 1975, Hollingsworth had owned the sign company with the most recognized billboard in Georgia—the one just north of Cordele on I-75 with the words *Butt Naked* and an arrow pointing down to a little white building where a notorious strip joint had done a brisk business. The rumor not only had the Reverend owning the sign, but being the proprietor of that building.

Rabbi Nathan Kohen, spiritual head of the Fitzgerald Hebrew Congregation during Sammy's youth, had been a kind man, but too strange for Sammy. Born in Latvia, the Rabbi had an accent so thick Sammy had never been really sure if he was speaking English or whatever language they spoke in Riga. The Rabbi had loved to talk about what the great Vilna Gaon had said about this and what Rabbi Menachem Mendel of Kotzk said about that. Sammy couldn't imagine that somebody would voluntarily spend his entire life studying the sayings of a bunch of bearded old men whose universe was the size of their little village or ghetto. He had watched his parents during services and noticed how intently they listened and how joyously they sang. To him, the whole thing had been a terrible waste of time.

After services, they would adjourn to the social hall, where Mrs. Moscowitz had filled the tables with food that would have made a congregation in Brooklyn proud: pickled herring, smoked kippers, gefilte fish, lox, bagels, and noodle kugel. Rabbi Kohen would approach the Lanskys, his mouth full of herring, sour cream sliding down his beard, and say, "Oiy, vat a beeg boy. God villing, you vill make your parents proud, no?" With that, he would pinch Sammy's cheek. Sammy, who by age ten had already grown a head taller than the Rabbi, had almost pinched him back several times.

To Sammy, religion was that part of his life that kept him different. Everyone else at the synagogue seemed to want to be different. They liked being Jewish, with all its strange, ancient customs; they enjoyed dancing the hora at weddings and singing Israeli folk songs. Louis Perlow, a Cordele merchant, loved it when Christians came to his house so he could explain the mezuzah, the little symbol above the door. When Sammy's friends came over, he would take them in the back door. That worked until his father came back from Atlanta with a mezuzah for that entrance as well. Then Sammy was forced to explain when asked, "What y'all got in them little boxes?"

♦ ♦ ♦

SAMMY DROPPED HIS PARENTS OFF AT THE CORNER of Magnolia and Lee and parked the car. There was a pretty good crowd today, so he had to park a street or two away. The synagogue was a two-story, red brick building that took up most of a block. It had been a Baptist church until 1940 when Moses Kaminsky, a merchant in Fitzgerald, had bought it. Sammy had heard this story over a thousand times. One day, in early 1940, Mr. Kaminsky told his brother, "I just bought a church, a Baptist church."

His brother, unpacking a new load of shoes, told him simply, "Good, Moishe, keep it."

Keep it he did. Mr. Kaminsky went to every Jew in this part of the rural Diaspora and convinced them all to make a contribution. By 1941, the church had become a synagogue. The inside had been shaped like a cross, so they turned the top part of the cross into a social hall. Each merchant donated a stained glass window. The Eternal Light, the light that sat atop the Ark and was never allowed to go out, was a gift from a synagogue in Atlanta.

"When Rabbi Kohen stood at the *bema* in 1941 and looked out at the fifty families of his congregation, tears rose in his eyes," Sammy's mother had reported. Of course, in 1941, she was on the other side of the world and might as well have been on another planet, but she recalled the moment fondly, nonetheless.

The sanctuary was small but beautiful. It was Wedgwood blue, deepened by the light passing through the ten stained-glass windows. There were three sets of pews going back fifteen deep. The rows on the right side facing the *bema*, or front stage, were by tacit agreement reserved for the Moscowitzes and their children, who now hailed from Atlanta, Birmingham, and Nashville. The *bema* had a lectern for the rabbi and one for the *chazzan*, or singer. The beloved Rabbi Kohen had died a number of years ago, so now the congregation—fifteen families—imported a rabbinical student from the Jewish Theological Seminary in New York once a month and for holidays. The *chazzan*, an eighth-grade-science teacher in rural Hahira, Georgia, was a heavily bearded man with a Crown Heights, New York accent. These two stood in front of the Ark—a small, free-standing closet on legs about three feet off the ground—where the Sefer Torah, or Five Books of Moses, was kept. The Ark was covered by a beautiful silk curtain with the words *Etz Chaim*, "Tree of Life," embroidered on it.

Sammy sat next to his parents just as the service was beginning. The service was not as long as it had seemed when Sammy was younger, but it was still too long for him. The constant standing and sitting drove him crazy. When the rabbi talked about the meaning of some ancient poem, Sammy looked at his watch. During the reading of the Torah, Sammy looked at his watch. During the sermon, Sammy looked at his watch. Finally, he could stand it no longer, so he walked out. His parents each gave him a look but said nothing.

He went to the side of the social hall and into the rooms where he had attended religious school. He looked at the pictures of confirmation classes and graduation classes on the wall. He saw Rachel's confirmation picture and thought she was just as pretty now as she had been at fifteen. There was no need to look for his picture.

He wandered into the small sanctuary where Junior Congregation had met—*had* being the operative word, since the decreased numbers left no need for this now. These days, the children ran about the main sanctuary. As he stared at the home of past Junior Congregations, Sammy sat in a chair and remembered this place thirty years before. He saw a young boy, about ten, carrying the Sefer Torah to the Ark. Suddenly, the little boy dropped the holy books. Mr. Steinberg, a local pawn shop operator who also served as director of education in the fifties, ran up and pushed the boy away, yelling at him, "In the days of the rabbis, you would have had to fast for forty days!"

All of the children stared at the little boy. He wanted to hide, but where? The synagogue was supposed to be a refuge, a safe haven from the isolation he felt being one of only a handful of Jews in the small town of Cordele. Wasn't this the place where his parents' broken English could be a symbol of survival? Sammy Lansky never found comfort here—not now, at age thirty-nine—and not when he had been the little boy who dropped the Sefer Torah.

"What did you think of Rabbi Sokoloff's sermon?" Frieda asked on the way back to Cordele after services.

"This boy, he is young," replied Nathan. "But he has the potential to be as good as the great Reb Peskin in Bialystok."

"Oiy! You always say that. This boy, I am sure, is one hundred times more of a mensch than that rebe of yours ever thought about being."

"Fruma, speaking such of the dead!" He spit on his fingers. *"Kain einorch!"*

"So what?" she said. "I met twenty Reb Peskins in the camps. They were all alike—praying and more praying. These big shot holy men in the old country hid behind their religion, if you ask me. They told us to pray when they should have told us to fight."

She spoke to Sammy, who was looking in the rear view mirror again. "People like your father, sometimes they forget how little good the praying did us."

Sammy interrupted. "Y'all want me to drop you by the store or take you home to get your car? Clete and I are gonna drive to Vienna to see some old buddies."

The Lanskys hated working on Saturday, but it was their busiest day. It was one of the compromises necessitated by living in America. In the old country, they'd never worked on Saturday. Of course, in the old country, they'd never had enough food, either.

"Gloria will bring us home from the store," said Frieda, referring to Gloria Boyd, who ran the store until they returned from services. "We do need for you to make a stop for us."

Sammy shook his head. He had seen his father take some books out of the synagogue's library. "Oh, jeez, more books for that weirdo. He still won't work or even drive on Saturday?"

"No," answered Nathan. "Bud Dee is a pious, wonderful man. Plus, he is the closest thing you have to a brother."

"Don't remind me," Sammy mumbled to himself.

Sammy left the interstate two exits before Cordele. He drove down Rock Top Road for about five miles, then turned onto a gravel and dirt driveway. They drove about a quarter of a mile, bouncing in and out of potholes the whole way.

"Why doesn't Buddy pave this driveway?" Sammy asked. "I'm going to have to get a front end alignment after this. Hell, I ought to send the crazy sonofa—uh, fool—the bill."

Finally, they entered a clearing and were greeted by a pack of at least ten scraggly dogs. At the end of the clearing was an old, cedar A-frame. Nathan hurried from the back seat, books in hand, and approached the house. Frieda asked her son to open the trunk, and when he did, she removed a small Styrofoam cooler and a woven basket. Sammy stood by the car, stretched and leaned on the Saab's roof.

As Nathan mounted the top step, a hulking figure appeared at the front door. Buddy Ambrose was Bigfoot. He stood six-foot-six and had the frame of a vault door. He was a thick-boned, square-jawed monster with black, shoulder-length hair, paws for hands, and eyes he usually hid behind sunglasses. Buddy had tattoos that could trigger nightmares. The dogs stopped their yapping one by one and sat down at their master's side, each jostling for a position closest to him.

"Bud Dee, Shabbat shalom," said Nathan, handing him the books. They shook hands. Frieda handed Buddy the basket and the cooler then disappeared in his hug. He looked in the basket and smiled.

Just what every south Georgia redneck wants, thought Sammy, *leftovers from a Sabbath dinner.*

"Why don't y'all come on in and set a spell, Mama and Papa L.?" said Buddy.

"We would love to, but we have to get to the store, and Sammy has to go visit his friends. Did you see Sammy, Bud Dee?" asked Frieda.

Buddy looked up and nodded in Sammy's direction. "Naw, reckon I didn't. How you doin', Sammy?"

Sammy waved. "Fine. Good to see you. You been all right?"

Buddy nodded. He took the books from Nathan. "I'll get these back to you soon. I 'preciate everything."

"We will see you on Monday," said Nathan. "Have a peaceful Shabbat." They waved good-bye to Buddy and left.

Sammy cursed under his breath as they bounced along the dirt road. "Yeah," he murmured to himself. "No wonder his brain's so jumbled, driving this road every day and all."

"He is truly a child of God," Nathan said as both he and Frieda shook their heads.

◆ ◆ ◆

BUDDY AMBROSE: THE PERSONIFICATION OF A DISCONNECT between what you see and what you get.

Every small town has its share of unusual people, and Buddy Ambrose played that role in Cordele. His daddy, tired of trying to make ends meet on a dirt farm in southwest Georgia, left when Buddy was eight. His mother was sure God was punishing her for some egregious wrong: It was bad enough to be poor, but to be poor, abandoned, and have a "slow" son was too much. Mama Ambrose took to religion in a big way, attending every tent revival within a hundred-mile radius. At first she took Buddy. Sometimes, however, the spirit would get her so worked up she'd find herself in the back of a bus with the preacher doing what they called the Lord's work. When Buddy asked about all the screaming, she stopped taking him.

He left school in eighth grade and drifted from one menial job to another. In 1962, he came to Cordele and was hired as a stock boy at Lanskys. At first, Nathan was afraid of Buddy. The boy said little, and when he did, his garbled and closed-mouth speech was hard to understand. But they needed help badly. For one year, Buddy came to work early every day, did his job well, got his paycheck, and went home. The Lanskys had no idea where he lived or what he did after work. His conversation was limited to the occasional yes, ma'am, or yes, sir.

One night as they were getting in their car, Nathan noticed a light in the storeroom where Buddy worked, and he mentioned it to Frieda.

"I wonder what Bud Dee is doing there?" she asked.

"Frieda, let us watch until the light goes out. Then we can go there and see if there is a clue. Yes?"

They waited in the alley off Tenth for one hour. Finally, the light went out and Buddy emerged from the building. When he was out of sight, they quietly entered the back room and flipped on the light. In the corner was a small table and chair. On the table was a paperback book called *A Life of Mitzvah: The Meaning of Being Jewish*.

"That is one of Sammy's Sunday school books," said Frieda.

"It appears that Bud Dee has been making better use of it than our Sammy ever did," Nathan observed, looking through the book.

During the next few weeks, Frieda and Nathan locked up the store every night and went across the street to Cindy's parking lot. Each night they noticed the light, and an hour later, Buddy would leave. The ritual continued for two weeks, but it was not always the same book. After *Mitzvah*, Buddy studied *The Five Books of Moses—The Lessons of Life*, and *What Is a Jew?* All were Sammy's unread books.

"What is going on here, I wonder?" asked Frieda one night.

"Maybe," Nathan replied, "maybe we should ask Bud Dee, or better yet," he said with a smile, "we will let Bud Dee tell us."

"How is that?" she asked.

Nathan took her by the arm and led her down the stairs. "This I will show you."

That night, after they closed the store, Nathan placed a copy of *Choosing To Be a Jew* on Buddy's desk.

For three nights after they placed the book on his desk, Buddy didn't go into his "study." He came to work and stayed to himself. On the fourth night, as they were closing, Buddy approached the Lanskys.

"I didn't take no books," Buddy said in a low mumble, his eyes on the floor. "Sammy give 'em to me before he left for college. I just wanted to read 'em." Buddy didn't look up or ever make eye contact.

Frieda studied him. He really did look prehistoric—hunched over, gazing at the floor. She stood on her tiptoes, placed her hand under Buddy's chin, and raised his head.

"You have no reason to look at the ground, Bud Dee. We are standing in front of you as friends." Frieda turned to Nathan, who nodded in agreement. "We are not on the ground, so please look up at us."

Buddy's head dropped as soon as she let go of his chin. Frieda reached for his chin again, but this time Buddy raised his head by himself.

"I, uh . . . I, uh, wanna, uh. . . ," he said in a low voice.

"There is no one here but us, Bud Dee. You can say what you want," said Frieda.

"I wanna be like you and Mr. L."

"You mean you should have your own store?" asked Nathan.

"Naw, not that. I like my job and all. It's about the best job I ever done had. Naw, I wanna become a . . ." Buddy hesitated, then finally got the words out: "I wanna be a Jew."

The Lanskys were stunned. "Sit down, son," said Nathan. "We should talk." The three sat in the storeroom and Nathan spoke. "Now, tell me why you want such a thing, Bud Dee."

"It's the way you and Mrs. L. treat people," Buddy said. "You know, fair and all. Y'all seem to have the spirit in you Mama's always lookin' for in them tent preachin's. I tole Sammy about it. He done give me these books to study. Said he never had no use for 'em."

Frieda moved her chair closer to Buddy. "You mean you want to become Jewish? To convert?"

"Yes, ma'am," he said, nodding his head but not changing his facial expression.

With those two words, one of the strangest occurrences in the four-thousand-year history of the Hebrew people was about to begin. Buddy Joe Ambrose was going to become a Jew. At first, Rabbi Kohen in Fitzgerald said no. He agreed only after he was convinced that Nathan would assume the major role in the process. Twice a week, Buddy would have dinner with the Lanskys. At first they discussed the history of Judaism, then the prayers. Nathan was amazed at how quickly Buddy learned to read Hebrew.

Nathan worked with Buddy for three years. In February of 1966, Buddy was given the Hebrew name of Bezalel in front of a full house at the Fitzgerald Hebrew Congregation, proving forever that truth is stranger than fiction.

CHAPTER SEVEN

After delivering the books and lunch to Buddy, Sammy dropped his parents off at the store. He parked for a minute to say hello to Gloria Boyd, then drove the six blocks to his parents' house. As he approached, he noticed a red Chevy pickup parked in the driveway. A chubby, bald fellow stood by the truck, hitching up his pants, grinning from ear to ear.

"Well, if it isn't Mister Big Shot Doctor, the Grand Potentate of All Pecker Checkers," said the man by the truck, "come home to see his lowly-ass subjects."

Sammy pulled up beside him. "You need some kind of rug, Clete. No wonder you're getting dumber: your brains are seeping out of your head. I thought you rednecks had extra-thick skulls to prevent that."

Clete rubbed his head. "She-it, rugs are for your house. Country boys don't wear no wigs."

After Sammy uncurled himself from the car, he and Clete hugged. Clete, who was built like a fireplug and came up to Sammy's chest, looked in Sammy's car.

"Where's Rachel? Spending the day in Fitzgerald to visit some folks, tend to her parents' graves?"

Sammy hesitated for a second. "Uh, yeah . . . she'll be coming here later."

"Damn, I was hoping she'd bring me some of that ruggee stuff she makes. Damn, that shit's good."

"It's ruggala, you dummy," Sammy said. He rubbed Clete's head. "You got to be Jewish to eat it now. The Rabbinical Council of North and South America, Brooklyn, and Unadilla declared it off-limits to rednecks last week. You boys gonna have to learn to live without it. Of course," Sammy said with a sly smile, "you could convert."

"Yeah, uh," Clete replied, adjusting his pants around his waist, "that's been done before down here."

"Just saw him. What a piece of work," Sammy said.

"Let's get going," said Clete, slapping Sammy on the back and pushing him toward his pickup. "Stewball and the boys are waiting for us, and they'll think we're some sort of city faggots if we drive up in that fancy foreign car of yours."

"Yeah," Sammy said, pointing at Clete's red Ford F-150, "but we'll have every redneck from here to Vienna waving at us in this damn thing."

The two hopped into Clete's pickup and headed north on Highway 41 toward Vienna, Georgia, where their friend Ray "Stewball" Barnes had a large feed-and-seed business. Barnes had gotten that nickname sometime after his birth and before his first birthday—nobody could remember exactly when or, for that matter, how the name came into being. Stewball and his wife had built their dream home on thirty acres between Vienna and Drayton along the Flint River. The house, with its thousand-square-foot basement, had become a haven for Sammy's old friends—a place to play pool, drink beer, and tell tales without interruption.

"How things going?" asked Clete after he had backed out of the Lansky's yard and headed out of town.

Sammy didn't say anything. He was staring at the tracks of the G. S. & F. Railway that paralleled the highway to Unadilla.

"What? You in a trance, son?" Clete asked, rolling down his window.

"Naw, I was just thinking about a couple of things," Sammy replied. "Remember how we used to come this way on our bikes, watch the trains go by? Think I learned more geography from the sides of those cars than I ever did in Mrs. Colley's class."

"Think watching them trains is what made you wanna leave Cordele?" Clete asked.

"Naw," Sammy replied then turned toward Clete. "I needed to get out, see the world. Find out where I really fit."

"She-it." Clete hit the steering wheel. "That place ain't nowhere on this planet. Everyone knows you was standing in the back of the line when they handed out normality. Hell, look at what you chose as your life's work—fooling with men's peckers."

"I told you why I picked urology. Everybody knows urologists are the smartest doctors around. Most of the folks we treat are cured of whatever ails them—during regular hours I might add—and nobody else is trying to horn in on our territory. I mean, the general surgeons and the chest surgeons are always having turf battles; the plastic surgeons hate the ear, nose, and throat docs; the neurosurgeons can't mention the orthopods without puking; and everybody hates the neurosurgeons, including their wives, because they're such assholes. We've got it made."

Clete laughed and thumped his belly. "Selling Hostess Ho-Ho's, Twinkies, and gas sounds a helluva lot easier and more civilized to me."

They rode in silence for a moment. "How's business?" asked Sammy, knowing Clete always said business was good, and it was. He owned five convenience stores in and around Cordele. It amazed Sammy that although he had been at the top of their high school class and Clete had been the anchor, Sammy was just starting to catch up to Clete financially.

"Going great," Clete replied. "Gonna buy a store off the highway in Hawkinsville in the next few weeks."

"And Rayann?"

"Fine. Gone back to work now that them young 'uns are at the university in Athens. Can you believe I got me two kids in college? Me, who barely got out of Crisp County High."

"Yeah," Sammy answered. "But I also believe in aliens and the tooth fairy."

Clete turned to Sammy and, with a smile on his face, made an obscene gesture with his finger. They listened to the radio and jostled with each other verbally for the next few miles until Clete pulled into Stewball's driveway. There were a number of cars and trucks almost filling the front yard. Clete parked, and the two descended into the party room after saying hello to Stewball's wife, Jewellette. Here there were a dozen or so of Sammy's oldest and dearest friends, all of whom began whistling and doing cat calls when they saw him enter.

Clete high-fived a few of his buddies and headed toward the bar. "Ol' Sammy Lansky comes home, and the entire male population of the Crisp County High School Class of 1964 shows up," said Clete.

"Hell, not the entire class," Sammy yelled to his buddy, who was now halfway across the room. "This is a very select group—these are the ones who can read and write, not one or the other."

Everyone laughed, then Stewball Barnes, who had reminded Sammy of Ichabod Crane when they were kids and still bore a distinct resemblance to him, raised his beer and said, "I'd like to propose a toast."

The assembled raised their beers and yelled, "Yeah!"

Stewball cleared his throat and, with his protuberant Adams apple bobbing up and down, began. "To our buddy, our friend, Sammy Schimi . . . Schimi-mule Lansky . . ."

"Stick with English, you idiot." Sammy gave his friend a punch. "Yiddish is for people whose family tree has branches."

The crowd howled. "Let me finish, you citified smart ass," Stewball said. "As I was saying, I'd like to propose a toast to Sam-u-el Lansky, the man who's done more than chicken shit, watermelons, and peanuts to put Cordele, Gee Ay, on the map." He raised his beer higher, and the crowd cheered.

Sammy raised his hand again. "Don't you guys have anything better than that cow piss?" Sammy said, referring to the beer Stewball had used to salute him.

Luther "Big Boy" Bates, who ran a backhoe service south of Cordele, hiked up his Sansabelt polyester pants and whistled to get everyone's attention. Big Boy was six-two, weighed close to three hundred pounds, and had played football at Troy State in Alabama—so getting people's attention was not a problem for him.

"Gentlemen," Big Boy said, clearing his throat. "Will someone please get this man a beer he can drink, so I can toast him?"

"Toast him?" Stewball asked.

Big Boy cut a look toward Stewball, then laughed. "Propose a toast. When did you get to be so goddamn proper?"

Clete reached in the refrigerator and found a Budweiser in the back. He handed it to Sammy, and Big Boy continued. "A toast for Sammy Lansky!" Everyone raised their beers. "To a man who used to get more ass than a toilet seat, but decided to go into a field where all the docs—" Big Boy started to laugh uncontrollably but managed to blurt, "Are queers!"

The toast brought down the house. Sammy shook his head and called for quiet. "I'd like to propose a toast," he yelled. "This is for me having enough sense to get the hell out of Cordele and away from you derelicts."

They spent the next few hours drinking beer and catching up. Just before four, Sammy and Clete said goodbye and hopped into the pickup for the trip home. Clete rubbed his belly and belched as he shifted the truck into reverse. He rolled the window down and waved goodbye one last time to Stewball and Jewellette, who were standing in their doorway. As they drove off, Clete rolled the window down some more and hung his arm out.

"Well, great party, huh?" Clete said, looking over at Sammy. "I don't care what you think. This is your home. You ain't never met nor gonna meet buddies like you got here, Sammy."

Sammy nodded and smiled. "Yeah, I'd have to live in the zoo to meet a crowd so interesting. That's for sure."

They bounded onto the asphalt and Clete belched again. "Me and Rayann, we figured you and Rachel might want to join us for dinner—new place just north of town called Vickery's."

Sammy was silent as he stared out of his window.

Clete waited a moment, then turned off the radio. "Where's Rachel, son?" He hit the steering wheel. "Damn, I shoulda known there was something going on when I asked you that back at Mama and Papa's house. Y'all have some falling out?"

Sammy turned to face his friend, shook his head, then looked back out the window.

Clete pulled onto the side of the road and put his car in neutral. "We ain't going no farther till I get an answer." He rapped on Sammy's arm. "You may be able to pull this silent treatment crap on some people, but me and you is more than good friends, so turn your ass around here, face me, and tell me what the hell is going on."

Sammy sighed, then turned toward his friend. "They still got a public park at the top of Lake Blackshear?" he asked.

"Yeah, picnic tables and some walking trails. Why?" asked Clete. "And what's that got to do with Rachel?"

"Stop there," Sammy said. "We've got to talk before we get home."

Clete stared at Sammy again with a curious look. "You ain't into nothing kinky, like shagging sheep, are you?"

Sammy hit Clete's forehead. "Just go to the park, you dumb ass."

They pulled into the parking lot, which was almost full. A woman stood at the public boat ramp frantically trying to keep her husband from knocking over a bank of trash cans as he tried to back their boat trailer into the water. Clete parked, and as he and Sammy met at the front of the truck, they heard a woman yell, "Cletis Towns! Well, how you been?"

Clete peered over to the table where the woman sat. She was well overweight and had wild, scraggly hair. "Well, hey, Becky, how you doin'?" he asked as he walked over to the table.

Sammy followed him and saw the woman, three other adults, and four children of various ages seated around the wooden picnic table. The table was full of plastic quart containers of soft drinks, bags of pork rinds and potato chips, and packages of Moon Pies. One of the other women was spreading paper plates around while a man grilled hot dogs and hamburgers.

"Y'all want something cool to drink?" the woman named Becky asked. "We got, uh, RCs and Co'Colas." Without waiting for an answer, Becky said to the man next to her, "Ricky, you know Cletis Towns. He owns that gas station over off 75 near Unadilla." She turned to Clete. "This here's my husband, Ricky."

The man named Ricky tipped his hat but didn't say anything.

Clete extended his hand, and the man took it. "Becky, you remember Sammy Lansky, don't you?" Clete said, pointing to Sammy.

She looked at him, then smiled. "My God, whatever happened? . . . Sammy Lansky, of course. You was in Clete's class at Crisp County. I was Becky Treadway, class of '66, two years behind you." She introduced Sammy and Clete to her husband and friends, not taking her eyes off Sammy as she did. "What you boys doing out here?" Becky asked.

Clete shrugged. "Taking a walk. Sammy's in town for the weekend. Just went by the Barnes' place for a while and decided to stop for a little walk before heading back to Cordele."

"Better get you some of this stuff," Ricky said, pulling some Backwoods Off! out of a bag. He opened his mouth very little when he spoke because there was a toothpick between his teeth at all times. "Them skeeters is still sleeping, but the no-see-ums is heavy."

Sammy and Clete thanked Ricky. Sammy doused himself, but before applying the spray, Clete walked back to the truck, removed his polo shirt and put on a T-shirt. He approached Sammy, who was still getting reacquainted with Becky. "Rayann'd kill me if I got my new shirt all sweaty," he said to Sammy.

They told the picnickers goodbye and walked down toward one of the streams that fed the lake.

"Hard to believe that's Becky Treadway," Sammy said in a soft voice. "She used to be one fine-looking woman. Had a set on her in high school. Wow."

"Yeah, amazing what four lousy marriages to four different losers will do to a woman." Clete said, wiping some of the spray off his face. "But I don't think we're here to talk about Becky."

"You're right," Sammy said. They were silent for a moment. Sammy took a deep breath, then spoke. "Rachel and I . . . are . . . have separated."

"Damn," Clete said in a much softer voice than was his usual. "When'd this happen?"

Some kids were skipping rocks in the stream, so Sammy held his thought. After they walked past, he spoke. "We split—that is, she left—last weekend."

Clete wiped his face with the end of his shirt. "Where's she gone? Fitzgerald?"

Sammy shook his head. "No, she couldn't do that. She's still teaching in Atlanta. She moved in with Joan Moscowitz temporarily."

Clete whistled. "You mean that girl from Unadilla? Daddy runs the big store there?"

Sammy nodded.

Clete stood, shaking his head and raising his voice slightly. "Ain't she the one who looks like she done been prepared by a mortician—all pasty faced with long black hair?"

Sammy looked up at his friend and smiled slightly. "That's her."

"I'll be goddamned if I'd spend one night in the same house as that woman. Hell, you'd wake up and think you'd been funeralized."

Sammy smiled. "You'd never wake up, because you'd never sleep with her running her mouth all the time. Anyway," Sammy said, putting his arm on Clete's shoulder, "I love Rachel, but we've sort of grown apart. We don't want the same things anymore."

A deer scampered about in the deep woods as they got closer to the lake. "She wants a baby and you don't—that right?" Clete asked.

"Babies aren't an issue now."

"Then what the hell is?" asked Clete. He went over to the lake and threw some water on his face. "I mean, you say she walked out on your ass. Rachel ain't the kind of woman to do that without a damn good reason. So far, Sammy boy, I ain't heard the reason."

Sammy raised his voice. "I told you we want different things from life now. She's—I don't know, sort of content with the way things are. I'm not. I want more, a lot more."

Clete spit on the ground and sat on a granite outcropping by the lake. "What's this new wool's name—Sally, Muffy, Tammy, what?"

"What are you talking about? There's no other woman."

"Ah, c'mon. This here is Clete you're talking to. I may have been born at night, but it wasn't last night. You been in heat ever since you got pubic hair. Some new wool cast her spell on you and *boom!* Out goes your beautiful wife."

Sammy crawled up on top of the granite. "There's no other woman—I'd write that down for you, but there may be too many big words in the sentence."

Clete removed his shirt and wiped his entire face and head. He stared at his friend for a few seconds. "You promise."

Sammy nodded.

"When are you two gonna get back together?" Clete asked in a soft voice.

"I don't know. I wasn't the one who left."

"Well, if I were you, I'd find out when Elvira's going out of town and I'd go over there and beg Rachel to come back. Anyway," he said as he started to put his shirt back over his head, "she ain't coming back while we're sitting here being attacked by these damn bugs, so let's go. Rayann'll be wondering where I am."

Clete finished putting on his shirt and began walking toward the truck.

"I did meet," Sammy said quietly, "an incredible woman."

Clete stopped dead in his tracks and turned around to face Sammy. "I knew it, " Clete said, snapping his fingers. "I knew Rachel wouldn't leave unless things were terrible. Me and you is like brothers. I can read you like a book. Who is this woman?"

Sammy shook his head. "I've only met her once—at a party. I shouldn't have said anything to you. It's just that after so many years of marriage it felt kind of nice for a woman, particularly such a beautiful woman, to sort of hit on me, that's all. Tell you the truth, if you hadn't mentioned the possibility of another woman, I wouldn't have even thought about it."

He stood and motioned for Clete to walk with him. "She was very nice, gave me her card, that's all. I've never . . . I mean, we've never been out on a date or even talked on the phone. Besides, someone that luscious probably has a husband and three boyfriends."

They walked for a moment in silence, then Clete laughed smugly. "Who she look like, Marilyn Monroe?"

"Marlene Dietrich."

"Look, I don't know no woman named Dietrich, but I do know you got yourself one of the most beautiful and smartest women that was ever born in Ben Hill County, and you'd be a fool to let her go."

"Yeah, I know, Clete, but how often does a goddess make a move on you when you're middle aged?"

They reached the truck. "Sammy, no goddess never made no move on me when I was no age. But I got me a good wife and some fine young 'uns and I got one thing you ain't never had in your whole entire life—I got me peace of mind.

CHAPTER EIGHT

THE NEXT MORNING, SAMMY HAD BREAKFAST with his parents at home. Sunday was their only respite from work, and it was a day of great importance to Frieda and Nathan. The afternoon and evening were for catching up on household chores, visiting the sick in the local hospital or stopping by to see friends at home. The morning, however, was a Lansky tradition: lox, smoked kippers, bagels, the Sunday *New York Times*, the Yiddish newspaper *The Forward*, and fellowship. The pungent odor of the smoked whitefish was always so strong and permeated the house to such a degree Sammy had learned to wear an old T-shirt and scrub pants at breakfast so his clothes wouldn't smell like a fishmonger's the rest of the day.

"So." His father placed three of the kippers on his plate. "You had dinner with Cletis and Rayann last night, no?"

Sammy looked at his father, who stared at the malodorous fish with delight in his eyes. "No, went over to Albany with some friends. Some new place called Vickery's, I think." Sammy buried his head in the sports pages of the Atlanta paper as he spoke. He knew from years of experience that his father could tell he was lying, almost like his nose began to grow. He had wandered around Cordele by himself thinking about his discussion with Clete.

Frieda entered the breakfast nook from the kitchen with a whole tray of freshly heated bagels. "Ooh, they smell so good, Mama," Nathan said. "Where are they from—that new bagel place in Albany? What they call it, Bagel Nation?"

Frieda put the tray on the table and wiped her hands on her apron. "What are you talking? You think I'm crazy? Bagel Nation—what is this name? Either you make the bagels at home or you buy them in a Yiddisha bakery. I could make them like my mother, *oleho hasholem,* did, but we," she said, looking up at Nathan, "we have a need to eat the rest of the week, too. So . . ." She sat down, putting two bagels on Sammy's plate. "So, I work during the week, and when Mrs. Moscowitz visits her daughter in Atlanta, she goes to Goldberg's Deli and buys bagels for me."

Sammy was still buried in the paper, so his mother spread cream cheese on his bagels and filled both of them with lox, tomatoes, and onions.

Nathan wiped his mouth and said, "What's the matter with the name Bagel Nation? To me, it's a compliment to our heritage."

Sammy looked up from the paper at his father and said, "Bagel Nation. How's that a compliment?"

"Oiy, don't ask," said Frieda, hitting her forehead with her hands. "We will spend the entire morning on a history of how the Jews and the Turks invented the bagel and almost all the other foods eaten in the world today. Then from there we will go to the glorious history of the relationship between the Turks and the Jews, and where it will end up, nobody knows." She pointed to Sammy's plate. "Eat your bagel before it gets cold, Schmuel."

Sammy took a large bite of the bagel and chewed slowly.

After an hour of talking about his old friends, Sammy went to his room, packed his bag, and prepared to leave. He hugged his parents at the front door, putting his long arms around both of them as he had done for so many partings.

Frieda backed away from him and wiped a tear from her eye. "If, by chance, you happen to see our Rachel . . ."

Sammy put his hand in the air to stop her. "I *will* see her, and I *will* give her your love." He looked from his mother to his father.

Frieda and Nathan looked at each other, then nodded. Sammy bent down, kissed both of them on the cheek, then went to his car.

The family home in Cordele was like a moral magnet to Sammy. When he was there under his parents' roof, the universe had a certain order to it. He didn't necessarily subscribe to that order and, for much of his life, he had fought it, but when he needed a moral hitching post, the red brick rancher with its two diminutive occupants was it.

The drive back to Atlanta was torture, not because of the overturned truck outside of Macon or the traffic for miles in either direction near the Atlanta International Raceway, but because nothing was right. He was on top of the world but felt as if the world was on top of him like a full-grown elephant. Rachel was gone, Clete was angry, his parents were disappointed, the only person who thought he hung the moon was Mo, and at this point that seemed as relevant as whether or not he used two-ply or four-ply toilet tissue. The only way to right the ship was to get Rachel back, and the only way to do that was to confront Mo and get some answers. Trouble was, he didn't want answers. He wanted to keep getting big checks so he could buy a lot of things like Mo and Sylvia. For over one hundred years, his ancestors in Europe had called America the Golden Medina and said the streets were paved with gold. He had a golden highway right in front of him, and nothing was going to mess that up. Or was it?

He arrived back at the house of mirrors and called Rachel. He told her about his parents and the boys at Stewball's, neglecting to say anything about his little walk with Clete.

"So," she said after all of the reporting had been done, "any word from our dear friend, Mo Gordon?"

Sammy twirled the phone cord with his fingers and hesitated. "Uh, haven't . . . uh, had the, um, chance to talk to him yet."

"Got the chance now?" Rachel shot back as if she had her lines right in front of her. "You know he's around since he's on call."

Sammy was silent. He could call Mo right after he hung up with Rachel and get this whole thing settled, or he could stew about it and feel like Atlas with the world on his shoulders. He could drive back to Cordele and pretend he was in a time machine—it was 1964, he was a big shot senior at Crisp County High and the whole world assembled itself on a big silver platter just for the pleasure of one Sammy Lansky. Trouble was, this wasn't some damn movie. This was live in Atlanta, and he didn't like the way the script was unfolding.

"I'll think about it and call him this week," he said in a quiet voice.

"Call me when you do," she shot back. "Don't call me if you don't."

For the rest of the week, Sammy thought about Rachel's concerns. He didn't call because Rachel always meant what she said. Her words about being a rainbow missing a few colors and why anyone would pay him so much money to be on a board went around in his head like the chorus of a catchy yet irritating song. Rachel and he had different views on money and life in general—they always had—but she would never leave him as long as he let her love him. The only thing that would force the life out of that love would be if she no longer respected him.

Prior to leaving his office Tuesday night, Sammy opened his filing cabinet and looked around for the *Georgia Stone* papers he had signed over a year ago. After scattering various documents on the floor in his office, he discovered an unmarked folder. Inside it were the papers he'd been trying to find. He read the legalese but to no avail. His father had said there were only two languages spoken all over the world, yet neither was an official language of any country—

Yiddish and legalese. He searched the document until he found what he was looking for:

> Paragraph 5. Ownership.
>
> Ownership of The Georgia Stone Institute shall at all times be by the shareholders. No control can be assumed by another party without the majority vote of the shareholders. Percent ownership is based as above in Paragraph 4 (Compensation) on one's equity, not on one's participation. That equity is wholly related to number of shares owned.
>
> All monies accrued as excess shall be distributed on a regular basis to be determined by the Board of Directors.

Sammy read the paragraph several times. He tried to make himself read every word, but the words ran together as if the ink had never dried. Unfortunately, he didn't see anything that would explain his recent good fortune.

Placing the papers back into the folder, he rose and looked out the window onto the sprawling city. He would call Mo tomorrow. Everything would be okay.

◆ ◆ ◆

THE NEXT AFTERNOON, SAMMY ARRIVED AT THE OFFICE an hour late. Surgery had taken longer than expected, and when he opened the door, his nurse gave him the "hurry up" signal. There was one thing he had to do before seeing patients.

"May-ree, could you get Dr. Gordon on the phone?" he said into the intercom.

"Sure, sir," Mary said loudly.

Moments later, Sammy heard the banging of the lithotriptor in the background as Mo came on the line.

"Hi, Sammy. What's up?" Mo yelled above the sound of the machine. "Wait a minute, Sammy . . . try to strap him down a little tighter. That ought to work," Mo said to a technician in the lithotripsy room. "Okay, Sammy, what do you need?"

"Done a lot of cases today?" Sammy asked.

"Hell, there're twelve on the schedule," Mo replied. "I'm on my fifth. Get a break after this one—Mitchell's got a case—then I got one more. That sound you hear is the cha-ching of the cash register. We're getting richer as we speak."

"When you think you'll be through?" Sammy asked.

"Well, let's see, it's two now. I'm almost finished. Mitchell will take a couple of hours to do his case—wish the bastard knew what he was doing—then I'll do my case. Ought to be finished by six or so. Why? Got something on your mind?"

"No, no, no. Just wanted to run something by you," Sammy said. "That's all."

Mo was silent for a second, and all Sammy could hear was the *bam bam* of the lithotriptor banging away like a sledge hammer on pavement. "Well, why don't you come by the house tonight? I'll show you my new toy and the plans for the addition. Sylvia is going to aerobics, so we'll be alone."

"Good. What time?" Sammy asked.

"How about seven-thirty or so? Sound okay?"

"See you then." Sammy looked up and saw his nurse pointing to a pile of charts in her hand.

◆ ◆ ◆

HE ARRIVED AT THE GORDONS' AT 7:15. Mo's chubby son answered the door and announced, "Dr. Lansky!" at the top of his lungs.

"Send him up!" Mo yelled back.

Sammy thanked the boy and went upstairs. Mo was in his opulent bedroom, which was easily a thousand square feet and looked like a bordello, only less refined. With all the loud, red velvet, it appeared Sylvia had decorated for Valentine's Day and never gotten around to removing the ornamentation.

Mo lay prone on a padded table getting a massage and a manicure. The masseuse was a tall, full-bodied blonde in her early twenties, who was sprayed into a white spandex body suit. The manicurist, sitting at Mo's fingertips, was a diminutive Asian woman covered by a bright, flowered smock.

"Sammy, how the hell are you?" Mo asked, looking up as Sammy entered the room. "This is my favorite form of exercise next to fucking. Oops, sorry, Mi." He looked at the attractive Asian manicurist, who continued her work unfazed. "I don't have to apologize to Crystal here," he said, turning his head sideways to see the masseuse. "She was thinking the same thing." Crystal smiled and winked at Sammy.

Mo put his head back on the table and said, "Finish up, girls. I've got business to discuss with my partner."

They nodded and within a few minutes were packing to leave. Mo got up and removed the sheet Crystal had wrapped around him. Completely nude, he ambled over to his chair, picked up his robe, and put it on. Men like Mo amazed Sammy. Here was this middle-aged, short, portly man with moles, warts and all the other excesses of one in his middle to late forties, parading around in front of two gorgeous women half his age, believing (or maybe pretending to believe) that they were interested in something other than his money.

Mo adjusted his robe then put his arm around Sammy. "Let's go into my study so we can talk in private."

Sammy had been in this mahogany-paneled room with its new, apparently untouched, volumes of Plato, Will Durant, Heine, and Churchill only once: when he'd signed his contract several years before. Mo had a stereo system that piped in classical music, and from his desk he could operate the stereo, lock all the room's doors, call every room in the house on the intercom, and talk on the phone—all with minimal effort.

"So," Mo began as he took a seat at his desk. "What's on your mind? Oh, before I forget, I meant what I said. You're now my partner." He rose and with a large smile, extended his hand to Sammy. "Henry's got the papers for you to sign. Said he'd be by the office in the morning."

"Thanks," Sammy said, still standing as he leaned over the desk and shook Mo's hand. "That's fantastic. I really appreciate the opportunity you've given me."

"You deserve it," Mo grinned. "God knows you deserve it. Well, what's on your mind, son?" Mo leaned back in his chair and motioned for Sammy to sit, which he did. "And, before you leave, remind me to show you my new toy."

Sammy squirmed in his seat for a second. "Uh, I've got to ask you a question or two about the lithotriptor. Tell you the truth, I wouldn't have given it a second thought had it not been for Rachel." He sat forward in his seat. "She kind of, uh, asked me a lot of questions I couldn't answer."

Mo sat up straight, placing his elbows on the table. "Rachel? I thought you two were kaput?" He thumped the fingers of his right hand on the desk.

"Well, we're what you might call temporarily separated." Sammy stopped and took a deep breath. "I mean, I don't . . . I mean,

I showed her the check for $940,000, and she didn't exactly understand what it represents and why the two different banks."

"Okay." Mo rested his chin on his clasped hands. "Go on. What else?"

Sammy adjusted himself in his seat. "It's confusing. I mean, I'm not sure how I earned such a large amount. That's what bothered her, uh, I mean Rachel, too."

Mo looked at him for a moment, shook his head, then started to speak, but held his thought. Again, he wiggled his fingers on his desk. "If you think Rachel is so smart," he said in a tone that was many shades darker than a minute before, "why are you two separated?" He stood up and leaned over his desk. "Seems to me that whatever you do with *us* is none of her business—particularly now. After all, I didn't just make her a partner. I didn't give her the opportunity to practice in the busiest hospital in Atlanta. I never signed any contract with her at all. My dealings have been with you, a board certified urologist, not your wife, who, if memory serves me correctly, is a grammar school teacher."

"Yeah, but, uh . . . "

"You got the check stubs?" Mo asked in a businesslike voice while extending his hand.

"Yeah, uh, sure," Sammy said, reaching into his pocket. "Got a copy of the checks, too."

Mo studied them for several seconds. "We use First Fulton because they're better at dealing with high-net-worth individuals." He walked to the bar behind Sammy's chair and poured a drink. His back was still to Sammy, so they were back to back when he said, "Don't blame you for your worries. This shit's so complicated, I think we ought to have Dellwood and Henry explain it to you."

He turned and walked past Sammy to his desk and sat on the front of it. "I apologize, but it's over my head." He tossed the tumbler full of light brown liquid down his throat and said with no enthusiasm, "To your health."

Mo was all smiles again, but it seemed to Sammy the only part of him smiling was his mouth. Mo slid off the front of his desk and got back in his chair. He opened the top drawer and retrieved a Daytimer. Thumbing through the pages, he looked at his schedule then up at Sammy. "I'll arrange a meeting. You don't worry about anything." He put the glass to his lips, realized it was empty, and got up to pour another.

"What are you doing for female companionship these days?" Mo asked from the bar.

Sammy turned around to face the bar. "Uh, nothing. I mean, I'm still married and all, like I said the separation is just, uh, a short-term type of thing."

"Married, schmarried," Mo said as he faced Sammy from the bar. "You're separated, which means you need a woman friend. I'll bet Sylvia can have one for you by ten tonight." Mo belt forth with a big faux laugh, then placed his drink on the bar, took Sammy by the arm and summarily escorted him downstairs to the front door, where they shook hands. Mo's palm was wet with sweat. Sammy didn't remember it ever being that way before.

"I'll have Sylvia call you," Mo said as he closed the door.

Sammy got in his car and drove off. First Fulton was a boutique bank used to dealing with big accounts. He had been stupid to listen to Rachel. Or had he? Mo had looked and acted like he'd been poisoned and the bad stuff had swamped his bloodstream when Sammy had asked about the big check. Truth is, Sammy had seen people who had been dead for several days look better than Mo had looked a few minutes ago.

Rachel's words to him were now almost two weeks old, but they were just as fresh in his mind as when they had been uttered.

He arrived at his apartment and, as he climbed the stairs to the bedroom, he realized Mo had not shown him his new toy and had not answered his question—where did the big check come from?

◆ ◆ ◆

MO WENT BACK UPSTAIRS AND SAT AT HIS DESK, trying to decide what to do. He reached for the phone twice and dialed a number but hung up before the call went through. He heard Sylvia drive up.

"Sylvia, can you come up to my office?" he said over the intercom system. "I've got to talk to you."

"Jesus H. Christ, I just walked in the goddamn door . . . wait a minute. Adam, get that stupid-ass dog out of here! I've told you a million times how expensive this kitchen floor is. What is it now, Mo?" she yelled into the intercom.

"Come upstairs. It's important."

"Let me get in the door all the way, for godsakes. Damn, nobody around here can wipe their ass without me."

Sylvia walked upstairs and entered Mo's office with a look of disgust on her face. She had on royal blue lycra exercise tights (which, for the most part, looked good on her other than a hint at saddlebags) and a lime green tank top that said, "Fit and a Hit." She dropped her exercise bag and put her hands on her hips. "What the hell do you want?"

"Sammy was here." Mo sat behind his desk massaging a drink. "He said Rachel was questioning the checks."

"Son of a bitch!" She slapped her thighs with her hands. "Since when did Mary Poppins get back into the damn picture? Goddammit! Have you told Mr. Big Stuff yet?"

"Just getting ready to do that now, wanted to tell you first." Mo spoke in a quiet voice. "You know, get your opinion."

"It's too late to get my opinion now, Mo Gordon. You should've listened to me a few years ago when you hired Gomer Pyle. If you remember, I told you they would be fine as domestics—put little uniforms on them, have them serve canapés at parties—but whatever you do, don't hire the bastard and his classless wife to practice with us. Now the bitch turns out to be his goddamn Mother Confessor." She shook her head and exhaled. "Well, you fucked up, not me, so call He Who Must Be Obeyed and see what he wants to do."

Mo squirmed in his desk chair. He started to dial the phone, then put it back down.

Sylvia grabbed the phone from him. "Goddamn, it's like having another child." She dialed Dellwood's number then handed the phone to Mo.

"Hi, Dellwood. Mo here."

"Mo, so good to hear from you. How are you?"

"Not good. Sammy just left here about twenty minutes ago. He wanted—or I should say his wife wanted—to know about the different checks."

Dellwood was silent for a second. "I thought you told me she was out of the picture."

"Yeah, uh, apparently he showed the checks to her before she left. I don't know how it happened, but she's got him asking questions."

"Well," Dellwood sighed. "What did you tell him?"

Mo, biting his lip, answered, "That we would meet and straighten everything out."

"Hmmm, what did he say then?"

"Nothing much," Mo said. "Seemed satisfied."

"Well, well, well. This *could* be trouble, but I've got a plan. Where is our boy now?"

"On the way home," Mo answered, taking a sip of his drink.

"What about wifey? Where is she?" Dellwood asked methodically.

Mo sighed. "Don't know for sure, but not living with him in their apartment."

"Good, good," said Dellwood. "That'll give us time to set things up. Sam may be a dumb shit, but he ain't dumb enough to want to go to prison for the next twenty years."

CHAPTER NINE 9

THE NEXT EVENING, SAMMY COULD HEAR THE PHONE ringing as he fumbled with his keys outside the front door of his apartment. He pushed the door open and managed to grab the phone just as the answering machine was picking up: "This is the Lanskys'. Sorry we're not . . ."

"Hello! Hello!" Sammy yelled into the machine, trying to interrupt it.

"Hallo," an accented voice said. "Dr. Sammy Lansky, please."

He was still breathing hard from his dash to the phone, so he waited a second to answer. He took a deep breath. "This is he."

"Hallo, Dr. Lansky. This is Rosvita Schuler. You met me a week or so ago at Dr. Gordon's house."

Sammy's breathing had slowed down, but now he could feel his heart pounding in his chest, and his shirt got as wet as if someone had hosed him down. Her melodious voice reminded him of her porcelain face. "Sure, sure. I remember. How, uh, are you?"

"Quite well, thank you. I know this is short notice, but I am nearby your house and was wondering if we might have dinner."

Sammy turned to look for a seat by the phone. He felt like Mo had looked the other night. He found a seat. "Uh, you mean tonight?" he asked.

"Why, yes. I am at Emory University, which I believe is quite close to you." Her voice was very smooth and professional.

Sammy bit his lower lip and wiped sweat off his forehead. "Uh, okay, I guess. Uh, look, since you're close, you may as well come by here for a drink, then we can decide where to go for dinner."

"Splendid. I will be there shortly. Bye-bye."

Sammy's hand was shaking as he put the phone down. He thought for a second, then rushed upstairs to clean up. As he was washing his face, he looked up and stared at his soap-laden image in the mirror. *How the hell did she know where I live?* he thought. He hesitated for a moment, then washed the soap off his face. *My address is not classified material,* he said to himself. *Certainly, she would have access to it through Georgia Stone.* He dried his face, brushed his teeth, then changed into a light green polo over which he threw a black sweater. He combed his hair while staring in the mirror. *Whoa,* he thought. *How the hell did she know I would be alone?* The doorbell rang.

"I'm coming," he yelled, checking himself once more in the bathroom mirror.

He bounded down the steps, took a deep breath and opened the door. "Hi, Ms. Schuler," he said.

She stood in the entranceway, smiling. "It's Rosvita, and may I call you Sammy?"

"Sure, sure." Sammy shook his head and cleared his throat. She looked at him just as she had at Mo's. He crossed his arms and tried not to stare at her.

"May I come inside?" she asked in a playful voice.

Sammy moved his head as if awakening from a trance. "Oh, sure, sure," he said, opening his arms and pointing inside. He watched her walk past him, trying not to make it too obvious he was gawking. She had on a black business dress that was cut above the knee and swooped down tastefully at the neckline. As she walked past him, he noticed that she was a muscular woman, yet feminine at the same time. He followed behind her, telling himself to look forward and not down at her legs.

"Have a seat, Ross-veetuh—is that how you say it?"

She sat on the edge of an upholstered chair and smiled. "Actually, the S is pronounced 'sh,' so it is 'Rosh-veetah.' "

Sammy, who was standing next to her, nodded. "I see."

"By the way," she said, motioning for Sammy to sit across from her, "I am sorry to hear that you and your wife are having some problems." She watched him sit. "Certainly, I hope everything will be fine."

Suddenly, his feeling of uneasiness had become one of curiosity. "How'd you know about that?"

She shrugged. "Dellwood, of course," she said. "I speak with him several times a week."

Sammy squirmed in his seat. He had told Mo, who must have told Dellwood, who, though it was none of his goddamn business, obviously had told the German beauty sitting in front of him. She did seem genuinely concerned.

"Who knows what'll happen?" He rose from his seat and opened his arms like a bird in flight. "Who knows? Anyway, would you like a drink?"

"Oh, yes. Vodka and tonic would be wonderful."

Sammy went upstairs to the kitchen, and while he did, Rosvita looked around the mirrored room.

"Hey, Ms. Sch—Rosvita, you want lemon or lime?" he shouted downstairs to her.

"Lime, please."

She wandered over to an old chest where there was a framed eight-by-ten of Sammy with a small man and woman. Rosvita smiled at Sammy's long hair, bell bottoms, and necklace. The couple with him looked Eastern European, almost Slavic. Next to this was a picture of Sammy and a striking, dark-haired woman she assumed was his wife. Rosvita looked at these photos for a moment, then she picked up a photo album, which she opened and began to thumb through.

Judging by Sammy's age, the photos seemed to be in reverse chronological order. There were pictures of Sammy and two people standing in the snow—a big Michigan Stadium sign loomed in the back. There were pictures of Sammy in full academic regalia, holding a diploma. There was another one in cap and gown, only Sammy was obviously younger. There were black and whites of Sammy on a bicycle, skinned knees and all, in front of a middle-class house.

"I'm coming, Rosvita," he called down to her. "I can't find the damn tonic. I think we've got some in the bottom of the pantry. Let me check."

Rosvita answered him and returned to the photo album. She was now much further back in time, and all the pictures were black and white five-by-sevens. In one photo, there was a place that looked like a concentration camp, but the buildings were made of what appeared to be canvas, and this place, with it's vegetation and sand, seemed to be tropical. There were no concrete walls like the ones she had seen at Auschwitz and Dachau—only barbed-wire fences. Just as she was about to turn the page, she noticed a faint inscription in the lower left corner of the photo. She removed the photo from the sleeve, and looked closely at the notation: *Cyprus 1947*.

She replaced the photo and turned the page. The next one showed hundreds, maybe thousands, of people on the deck of an old freighter. Every available square inch of the ship was covered with humanity—even the large smokestack. Many people waved handkerchiefs. On the side of the ship was a banner in English, which stretched for what she guessed was at least twenty-five meters. Rosvita could read this very well.

*We survived Hitler. Death is no stranger to us.
Nothing can keep us from our Jewish Homeland.
The Germans destroyed our families.
Please don't destroy our hope.*

The name of the ship, *Nishoma Yisroel*, followed on a separate sign.

Rosvita felt a tear fall on her hand, and she quickly wiped her eyes on her sleeve. Her body was trembling, and she felt faint. She took a deep breath, trying not to cry, but she was shaking so hard she found it difficult to hold the book of photos.

She started to close the album when she felt something under the last photo—it was another picture stuck to the one above it. She gently pulled the two apart and stared at the one on the bottom. What she saw made her chin quiver uncontrollably, and she began to sob softly and without interruption, her tears falling on the photo. There, standing on a dock in front of the same ship, was a youthful image of the two older people she had seen in the pictures with Sammy. They had a baby in their arms.

"Sorry it took so long," Sammy said as he entered the room with the drinks. "I must've had to go to the bathroom awful bad when I came home with this tonic. I finally found it in the bathtub along with a six-pack of beer."

Rosvita quickly put the album down and moved to the window—away from him—wiping her eyes again on her sleeve. She turned to look at Sammy, who held her drink out for her, and she began to cry.

"What's the problem?" he asked, screwing up his face and handing her the drink.

She shook her head and waved him off. "It is nothing really. Just that some of those photos . . . I mean, did this happen to your family?"

He nodded.

Suddenly, without even putting her drink down, Rosvita hugged Sammy, spilling some of her drink on his sweater, and squeezed him as she rocked back and forth, tears streaming down on his neck.

He stood with his arms by his side, drink in hand.

She backed away and began looking for a handkerchief in her purse. "I'm sorry, Sammy," she said, wiping her tears.

Sammy looked around for something to wipe her eyes but, unable to find anything suitable, gave her a cocktail napkin. Rosvita dabbed her tears. "I am okay now. It's just that those photos . . . they . . . well, I am German, and so embarrassed that this," she said apologetically and pointed to the album, "is part of my heritage. I am sorry, so terribly sorry." She wiped her eyes and nose. "Can we leave and go to dinner?"

"Okay," he said. "You sure you're all right?"

She smiled, wiped her eyes, and nodded.

The phone sitting next to his photo album rang. Sammy looked at it until it completed the second ring. The only person who would be calling him now was Rachel, so before the third ring ended and the answering machine picked up, he turned the volume down.

"I'll get it later," he said, opening the door for Rosvita.

They had dinner at one of the funky restaurants that lined Atlanta's Piedmont Park. The eatery known as The Prince of Wales had only one distinguishing feature: It offered outdoor dining right across from the park.

As they sat outside at their table, Rosvita seemed to be very interested in Sammy and asked him a lot of questions about his present life and his past. "So your parents, they are European?"

"Ex-European," he answered with a smile.

"The name Lansky, what country is this?" she asked. "It is not German. Maybe Polish, no?"

Sammy took a bite of his dinner. "Neither one. It's Jewish. But," he said as he wiped his mouth, "Lansky is sort of a made-up name anyway. My mom and dad changed it from Zychilinsky—Nachum and Fruma Zychilinsky became Nathan and Frieda Lansky." He smiled. "Still pretty ethnic, but not so harsh."

Rosvita tapped the side of her glass repeatedly with her index finger, then excused herself and went to the bathroom. When she returned, she took a sip of wine, then asked, "Were they . . ."

He shook his head and interrupted her. "Auschwitz, Class of 1945."

Rosvita looked down, closed her eyes, and sighed.

After dinner, they decided to take a walk in Piedmont Park. It was a clear but cool night. The path winding around the park was filled with pink and white dogwoods in full bloom, and the interior of the park was awash with red, white, and pink azaleas and purple rhododendron.

"What about you?" Sammy asked as he removed his sweater and offered it to her. "Lived in Germany all your life?"

She pulled it over her head and straightened out her hair. "No, not really." She adjusted the sweater to fit her torso as they walked past the old bathhouse. "I was born in a little village in what was then part of so-called Greater Germany, but now is Poland. My parents were killed at the end of the war."

Sammy stopped and looked at her. "Sorry," he whispered.

She smiled at him, put her arm inside his and guided him toward the lake. "I was very lucky. I lived in an orphanage outside of Brno in Czechoslovakia until 1948. When I was seven, a German family from a small village on Lake Constance adopted me. My adopted father was an engineer with MAN, which was headquartered near our village. Do you know MAN?"

Sammy shook his head.

"One of the largest manufacturers of buses and engines in Europe. I worked there, too, until this job with Dornier came along."

They walked along Lake Clara Meer, which formed the center of the park. "So how long have you been in Atlanta?" Sammy asked.

Two bicyclers sped past them, prompting Rosvita to nudge Sammy up off the paved path onto a gravel one. "Let's see," she said. "Off and on for several months, but now . . ." She squeezed his arm. "I think I will be here for a year or so.

"You are happy practicing with Dr. Gordon, I think?" she asked.

"Yeah, sure."

"The others, Dellwood and Henry, you like them, as well?"

Sammy hesitated, and she smiled and said, "You are different from them, particularly Dellwood, so you have reservations, maybe?" she said.

"Yeah, that's one way you could put it," he replied. "There are some things about him that . . ." Sammy shook his head. "Never mind."

"What were you going to say?" she asked.

"Nothing, nothing."

Sammy didn't want to get into Dellwood with her. After all, she did seem to have been somewhat cozy with him at Mo's party. Maybe she had even been his date. Sammy didn't know this woman well enough to risk saying something he might regret.

They came to a large swing that overlooked the lake next to an old bandstand that had been erected in the 1890s for the Southeastern Cotton Exposition. They swung in silence for a while, then talked about growing up. Rosvita told Sammy about skiing in

Garmisch and picnics on Lake Constance, and he had her in stitches with tales of his escapades as a youth in Cordele.

Around nine, they began to walk out of the park by way of the botanical gardens. Once again she put her arm inside his. They passed the greenhouse and reached a pond with a bank of hydrangeas along the edge.

"To me, these are the ugliest plants around," said Sammy. "I mean, look at those dead looking limbs just poking out from the root. I'd never plant them if I had a garden."

"Yes," she allowed. "But the hydrangeas are so beautiful in the summer and fall. Azaleas are green and full all year long, but they bloom for such a short time. It's almost like they tease you. But when the hydrangeas awaken, the ugly duckling becomes a swan for many months."

He shook his head. "I still wouldn't have them."

"They are also very adaptable, Sammy. You can take pink and red flowered ones, put them in acid soil, and they will turn blue or purple. On the other hand, they can be made to bloom a brilliant red just by adding lime to the ordinary red ones. Yet, despite these differences, brought on by changes in their surroundings, they are still hydrangeas."

She let go of his arm as they walked away from the bank, past the entrance to the park and toward Sammy's car.

"You know," she said, lowering her voice, "in a way, the Jews are like hydrangeas."

Sammy stopped on the sidewalk, a quizzical look on his face. "What?"

"They are. The Jews have adapted to life all over the world. Yet they hold on to the traditions and customs that make them Jewish."

He shook his head and gave her a dubious look.

"You," she said, pointing to him, "grew up in a small southern town, and other Jews grew up in New York City. I would think you have very little in common with them except for the fact that no matter what happens, you are still Jewish."

"Rosvita, where did you get this stuff? Did you think it up in the shower when you should have been singing?"

She laughed. "Seriously, the more I think about it, the more I believe I am right. Most hydrangeas flourish in warm weather but need to be in the shade. A few can stand direct sunlight. The European Jews like to be comfortable, so they keep a low profile, like the shade-lovers. The Americans . . . well, let's just say they like the limelight."

That night, Sammy lay in bed trying to figure out what had happened earlier that evening. Rosvita was truly one of the most captivating women he had ever met, but he was wary of her and, more important, he was married to Rachel. In truth, he missed his wife. Maybe Clete was right about him. Maybe he would never have peace of mind. Maybe he would never get it right.

◆ ◆ ◆

AT ABOUT THREE O'CLOCK IN THE MORNING, Sammy got up to get a glass of water. As he stood in the kitchen, he suddenly felt as if the walls were closing in on him. He began to sweat and feel light-headed. Images of Rachel, Rosvita, and Mo went round and round in his head. Rachel, Rosvita, and Mo chased each other one way then the next—a disturbing carousel. He had been an engineer before becoming a doctor, so he liked things to be in order, not chaotic as they were now.

Rachel was gone, for how long he didn't know. Rosvita had appeared—the timing was almost orchestrated. And Mo—why had Mo looked like a corpse when Sammy asked him about the checks? Yes, the walls were closing in on him, he was no longer in control, and that just wouldn't do.

CHAPTER TEN 10

S AMMY SAT IN HIS OFFICE THE NEXT MORNING, looking at his watch. It was 9:30, and his nurses hadn't brought back the first patient. *Here we go again,* he thought. *When we get a late start like this, it messes up the whole day.*

"May-ree," he called into the intercom. "What's going on? I know Mrs. Pottruck is supposed to be here for her post-op visit at nine." He looked at his watch again. "Here it is half-past, and I'm still sitting on my duff."

The silence told Sammy things might not be right. Mary was never silent. "Uh, sir," she started. "We, I mean, I was told to cancel your morning patients."

"What?!"

"Uh, yes, sir. Dr. Gordon told me yesterday that Mr. Dolt and his friend—you know, the tall gentleman with the beard—would be by for a meeting in the morning. He, Dr. G., that is, said you'd be expecting them." She cleared her throat. "I hope that's okay."

Sammy took a deep breath and squeezed the phone. "Sure, it's okay, Mary. Thanks."

Fifteen minutes later Dellwood Dole and Henry Morton knocked on Sammy's door.

"Sam," said Dellwood, extending his hand across Sammy's desk. "How *absolutely* wonderful to see you." Sammy kept his hands folded on top of his desk, so Dellwood reached across it to pat them. Sammy leaned back and crossed his arms.

Dellwood and Henry sat across from Sammy. Dellwood arranged himself in the chair and, as he examined his nails, said without looking up, "Henry, do you have something to say to Sam?"

Henry took some papers out of an expensive briefcase. With his mouth moving stiffly as though his jaws had been wired the day before, he said, "We owe you a bit of an apology, I think."

Sammy sat back in his small cloth desk chair and looked first at Henry, then Dellwood. He said nothing.

"Uh, ahem," Henry said, clearing his throat. "We're so sorry about the mix-up. It never should've happened. Just one of those things."

"It's just—it's just an abomination! That's what it is," said Dellwood, hitting Sammy's desk with his knuckles. "Personally and professionally, I'm so embarrassed. I feel like, oh, God, I don't know, nothing like this has *ever* happened." Dellwood had a pained look on his face.

Henry waited till he knew Dellwood was completely through with his playacting, then he chirped: "We need to arrange a meeting away from the hustle and bustle of your office, so that we can go over all the details and straighten this out. Meanwhile, to make things easier in the future, we've arranged for your checks to be deposited directly to the bank. All we need," he said as he laid the papers in his hand on Sammy's desk, "is for you to sign here and here." He pointed to the appropriate places. "This is for convenience, of course. A mere formality."

Sammy looked at the papers but said nothing. Now he could add these two to the list of runners using his brain as a track. Mo had apologized to him, and now these two had done the same—but for what?

Dellwood twisted his pinky ring and stared at Sammy. "You don't have to sign anything you don't want to, Sam." He stood and walked over to a bank of windows. "It's just that we think it would make things so much *simpler* for you." He turned back to face Sammy, then moved over to Sammy's desk and sat on the edge of it. He caught his own reflection in the framed poster above Sammy's head and adjusted his tie and smoothed his hair. Without saying anything, he stroked a paperweight for several seconds.

"Sam, we—Henry, Mo, and I—think you have a bright future in our organization. Now, you know I'm not a doctor and wouldn't know which part of a stethoscope is up or down." Henry simpered, as did Dellwood. "Not to mention some of these instruments of torture you urologists use." He and Henry chuckled. Sammy remained expressionless.

"It's sort of the same...," Henry began before he was given the signal to be quiet by Dellwood.

"Let *us* run the business." Dellwood pointed to himself and Henry, then reached across the table and patted Sammy's hand. "You stick to being a doctor."

Sammy wet his lips but said nothing.

"Well," Dellwood said, rising off the desk. "I hope you accept our apologies. Now if you will sign the direct deposit form, we can go."

Sammy looked at the form and the yellow places where he was supposed to sign, then at Dellwood. "I'd better have my lawyer look these over." He turned to Henry. "S. Alan Hamburger. I think you met him when I signed on with Mo."

"Yes, yes," chirped Henry. "He's competent counsel, of course, but I assure you these are merely vanilla forms that don't require his services."

Sammy nodded. "Let me run them by him." Sammy half-smiled. "After all, with the money we've made, whatever I spend on legal fees will be insignificant, won't it?"

Dellwood straightened his coat and patted Henry on the back. Henry rose, and Dellwood pushed him toward the door.

"Absolutely, my dear Sam," Dellwood said, his hand on the doorknob. "You get all the legal advice you need. After all, we were just trying to do you a favor." With that, he opened Sammy's door and pushed Henry out.

Sammy watched them walk down the hall, then moments later, he looked out his window and saw the two walking along the outside plaza to their car. He sat at his desk for a moment, then placed a call.

"Farnsworth Jay," a woman answered.

"Yes, I'd like to speak to Mr. Hamburger."

"Certainly. May I tell him who's calling?'

"Sammy Lansky, L-A-N-S-K-Y. "

"Just one second please, Mr. Lansky." As he waited for his lawyer to answer, Sammy prepared himself for the usual routine which, by normal human standards, was anything but normal nor usual. The attorney's seldom-used first name was Sigmund, and the boys had developed a greeting based on it.

"Alan Hamburger," a masculine voice said.

"Siggie."

"Sammy."

"Siggie."

"Sammy."

"How the hell are you, Siggie?"

"Sammy, if you'd seen who I woke up with this morning, you wouldn't even ask. Irene the Machine, that's what I call her. Luscious and lascivious. What a combo."

Siggie and Sammy had met at Emory when the two were studying, respectively, law and medicine. Siggie's brilliance as an attorney was surpassed only by his braggadocio as a ladies' man.

"I need to ask you some questions on the QT," Sammy said. "Maybe buy you dinner sometime soon."

"Ooh, I love intrigue. Buying me dinner will prove to be more expensive than you're used to, I'm afraid."

"I can handle it, particularly since I have no intention of paying you for your opinion. Remember, I was the one who introduced you to Candy Cane," said Sammy, referring to a stripper who'd been a patient and let it be known she was looking for some outside work.

"God, my pulse just went up to three hundred," Siggie responded. "Where's Candy keeping herself these days?"

"Don't know. Anyway, let me tell you what's on my mind." Sammy gave his friend a brief history of lithotripsy in Georgia. He told him about seeing the machine at the American Urological Association meeting in 1983 and how that had piqued his interest enough to go to Munich a few months later to visit the Grossharden Clinic, where it had been invented. He'd brought the idea home to Mo, who'd immediately gotten Dellwood and Henry involved. He ended by telling Siggie about Lithotripsy Associates, LithoServices, the two checks, and the two banks.

"Hmmm," Siggie said. "Sounds interesting. Let me make some notes. Just a sec." A moment later, Siggie got back on the phone. "So, they signed up a hundred docs and divvied up five hundred shares by giving the docs the right to purchase up to five shares each in Lithotripsy Associates. Right?"

"Yep," Sammy answered.

Siggie talked to himself for a second, then spoke into the phone. "Okay, so because you doctors were all part of this big group, you could treat Dr. Joe Blow's patient from Valdosta and the money went to Blow and not you."

"That's right, Siggie. Dole said it was perfectly legal."

Siggie hesitated and made a clucking noise with his tongue. "Think he's right about that." He was silent for a moment. This was no longer Siggie of Candy Cane fame; this was lawyer Siggie. "What exactly does this LithoServices do?" he asked.

"It was or is the management team led by Dellwood Dole. He organized the whole thing, bought the machine—using the doctors' money, of course—hired the personnel, did all the negotiations with the hospitals and the insurance companies, and now runs the day-to-day operations of the machine."

"What was Dole et al's stake in this whole thing? I mean, how were they to be paid?"

"Well, uh, Dole created this management team consisting of him, me, Mo, and Henry Morton—that's LithoServices I told you about. He said that since we were the general partners, we didn't have to buy any shares but would participate in the profits. Sound okay to you?"

Again Siggie said nothing, but merely made the clucking noise with his tongue. "Um, probably completely legal. Have you asked them, I mean this Dole guy, about the different amounts?"

"Not exactly. I asked Mo, and he said Dole would straighten it out."

"And?" Siggie asked.

"Dole and Morton came by the office just now. They were falling all over themselves with apologies."

"Apologies? For what?"

"I guess not explaining things to me. Tell you the truth, I really don't know."

Siggie went silent again, which made Sammy much more nervous than if he were talking as usual. Finally, he asked, "Any more checks since the last one, Sammy?"

"No, next one's due first of July. They want me to sign this direct deposit form—said it'd make it easier. I told them I'd have to show it to you first."

"Good work, good work. Got any records?"

"Yeah," Sammy replied. "Check stubs, documents I signed, things like that."

"Send them to me—better yet, bring them to me. Got time to do that?"

Sammy laughed sarcastically. "As a matter of fact, I've got all morning."

"I'll be here till noon. I'll look at them and call you tonight. See you soon," Siggie signed off.

"Thanks," Sammy said as he hung up.

◆ ◆ ◆

EARLY THAT EVENING, SAMMY SAT IN HIS APARTMENT, waiting for Siggie to call. The place seemed to be getting smaller and smaller, and he hated it. If Siggie had good news for him and everything was all right, the first thing he was going to do was call Rachel and demand they settle things and get back together. He knew he was incomplete without her, and she could breath some life into the apartment and him.

The phone rang, and he almost fell to the floor trying to get to it. "Hello," he said, trying to untangle the cord.

"Sammy."

"Hi, Siggie. Well? . . ."

"Who owns this machine?" Siggie asked in a voice that didn't give Sammy any comfort.

Sammy hesitated, and his voice cracked as he spoke. "The doctors."

"Huh. Who told you that?"

Sammy wiped sweat from his brow and paced with the phone in his hand. "What? Um, I'm not sure what you mean."

"Who told you? Or let me put this another way: Have you seen any documents that say you and the other doctors in Lithotripsy Associates own the machine?"

"I, uh . . ." Sammy was breathing rapidly, and he had to change hands with the phone because of his wet palms. "I guess. I mean that was the reason Lithotripsy Associates was set up—to own the machine, I think. In fact, I'm sure it was set up like that. I told you how it was done: Each doc had to put up a thousand bucks a share and sign a bank note for twenty-five grand a share to buy the thing. Dole and Morton took that money, bought the machine, paid for advertising, hired personnel, etcetera."

Siggie spoke in a solemn tone. "Sammy, everything I tell you is mere speculation on my part—your documents are very nonspecific—but here's what I think is going on. Lithotripsy Associates allows all one hundred urologists to act like a big group practice—that's why it's perfectly legal for you to treat one of your so-called partners' patients and have the money go to the referring doctor, who happens to be your partner in Lithotripsy Associates."

"Yeah, that was the idea behind it," Sammy said. "Dole said it would be worth it for me and Mo to do that because we would make extra money since we were also general partners."

"My question is where that *extra* money comes from."

Sammy hesitated. "I thought I'd mentioned that to you. The doctors get a fee for treating the patient, but there's a separate fee, billed to the insurance companies, for the use of the machine—it's called the technical fee."

"Is that where your $9,400 came from—the technical fee?"

So far, Sammy had no answers, only more confusion. "Yeah, that's right. What is this, Siggie's Socratic method? I need some answers, not more questions."

The lawyer began his annoying clucking sound again. "I can't prove this, but I think LithoServices owns the machine. I think they have a contract that none of you docs have ever seen."

"No way," Sammy said as he began to pace again. "When we set this up, Dole specifically said it was to be a doctor-owned machine."

Siggie scoffed. "And *I'm* telling you that I could fart right now and fly down the block. You guys had a great deal—the docs around the state could be doing a procedure in their hospital while you and Mo were making money for them in Atlanta. At the same time, you and Mo became known as the stone kings, so you had tons of your own patients. *Now*, the other ninety-eight guys are even more ecstatic because they just got checks on top of the money they've already made—particularly since they only had to sign guarantees for the machine, with very little out of pocket cash. They're happy, so why suspect that they're getting royally screwed by the management team, who's keeping the lion's share of the technical fee for themselves?"

"Oh, shit."

"Sammy, my old friend, I don't know exactly how these guys have done it, but I think your management team set up a scheme to defraud the urologists out of millions."

Sammy plopped down in his chair and closed his eyes. "Oh shit," he muttered. "They figured me and Mo wouldn't say anything. I mean, who would, since we'd be making over a million bucks?"

"That's just for this year. You could make enough money on this thing over the next few years so that you'd be set for life.

Particularly since you told me they are planning to move their operation into other states."

"Huh," Sammy whispered.

"There's one other thing, my friend. I just used the words *fraud* and *management team* in the same sentence." Siggie paused for a second.

"Yeah, so . . ."

"You are part of that team, and you have the money to prove it."

Sammy put his hands on his head, bent over, and began to rock back and forth. He started sweating as if he were in a steam bath. "Goddamn, Siggie! What the hell should I do? I'll—I'll give the money back. I'll go to the police, tell them everything!"

Siggie was as cool and calculating as his friend was distraught. "Don't do either one right now. Anyway, what would you tell the police? We don't know anything yet. Listen, after I read the documents, I called a criminal lawyer, Dudley Kessler—you remember him from Emory, everyone called him Dooge—he has agreed to use one of his PIs to look into the matter. He said he'd get in touch with you within a week."

Sammy tried to speak, but his throat was too dry.

"There's one other thing I need to tell you," Siggie said.

"What?"

"There's a very good chance what these guys have done is not fraudulent, not illegal, only highly unethical. If that's the case, then you have a decision to make—it may be hard to blow the whistle on a deal that's providing you with such a huge payoff and promises only to get bigger. I mean, you could retire in a few years. It could be a tougher decision than you think."

Sammy was silent for a moment, then said, "Thanks."

He rocked back and forth for several minutes, rubbing his eyes. He stood, took a deep breath, and decided to take a walk and consider his options. *If Siggie is right,* he thought, *Rachel was right.* He picked up the picture of his parents and him in front of Michigan Stadium and stared at it. How would he explain this to them? Their spirit was in him, but he had failed them terribly by rejecting their inner goodness. He replaced the picture and, in so doing, knocked over another one. His hand was shaking, so when he reached for the second photo, he inadvertently pushed it behind the chest. His hand was too large to remove the picture, so he moved the chest slightly and tried to retrieve the photo, and it fell to the floor as he did. Sammy bent down, picked it up and replaced it on the chest.

As he began to move the chest back into place, he realized something wasn't right. Wiping the sweat from his face, he bent down again—this time his heart was pounding so furiously that he had to sit on the floor. In front of him, behind the chest, was a white box that appeared to be a tape recorder. It was plugged into the lower half of a two-pronged phone jack with the phone itself plugged into the upper half. A wire from the recorder was inserted into a standard wall outlet.

Sammy touched it gingerly. Then he unplugged the phone jack connection and the wall outlet. He pushed a button and jumped back when he heard the conversation he had just had with Siggie. Beads of sweat formed on his face, and instantly his shirt was drenched. All life lines were gone, and now the vise was really closing in on him.

He closed his eyes and tried to organize his thoughts. *When did they do this? How did they do this? Who were "they"?*

He removed his shirt and used it to wipe his face. As he did this, the terrible truth hit him—*Now it all fits together,* he thought. He had come down from fixing drinks upstairs and found Rosvita at this very chest a few days ago. She just happened to know about Rachel's leaving, just happened to be in the neighborhood, just happened to want to get to know all about him, just happened to be Dellwood Dole's friend, and just happened to work for a company that stood to make many millions from its association with Dellwood and his docs.

Sammy ran upstairs and washed. He put on a new shirt, went downstairs, and picked up the phone. From his wallet, he removed the card Rosvita had given him. He dialed the first three digits, then stopped, looked at the phone and hung up. Moments later, he was in Emory village using a pay phone.

"Hallo," the lyrical voice said.

"Hi, is this Rosvita?"

"Yes, is that Sammy there?"

He was determined now. There would be no hesitation in his voice. "I need to see you tonight."

"Well, it's after seven. What time. . .?"

"Now."

Rosvita was silent for a second, then gave him directions to her house.

CHAPTER ELEVEN 11

Rosvita lived on the north side of town near Chastain Park, so Sammy had about a twenty-minute drive. He would try not to get emotional or too confrontational, but the more he thought about things, the greater his anxiety and the more accusatory his spirit became. He checked the directions over and over and drove past her house on Runnemede Road three times before he had the nerve to go down the short driveway. The house was a small brick ranch, and despite the onset of dusk, children of all ages played in two or three different yards.

He parked and began moving, step by nerve-wracking step, to her front door. *This must be what death row inmates feel like as they make that final walk,* he thought. *Difference is they kind of know what they are getting into.* He had promised himself he would use the same demeanor with her that Siggie had used with him: slow, monotonic, matter of fact. She was standing at the door as he approached.

"Hallo." She greeted him with a smile that looked painted on, like a clown's.

"Hi," he answered brusquely. "Let's go inside. I've got a few things to ask you." He pointed toward the inside of the house. The smile disappeared; her face was ashen.

He followed her into a small but airy den that had a high, vaulted ceiling, a fireplace, and a large, sliding glass door leading to the outside. The furniture was all light and contemporary, but right now the room was morgue-like.

"Have a seat, please," she said, offering him one of the two matching, cream-colored love seats. "Would you like something to drink?"

Sammy shook his head. She never took her eyes off him, and her mood mirrored his: she appeared ready to explode right through her skin. Her look made Sammy feel he was right about her, and that sickened and emboldened him at the same time. When he didn't sit, she spoke.

"Would you like to go outside? We could . . . we might . . . sit on the deck. It is quite nice."

Sammy nodded, and she opened the sliding glass door. Outside, she had a beautiful, sloping back yard with a deck extending out over at least a third of it. She sat in a wooden rocking chair, and he followed suit.

They rocked in silence for a moment, staring out toward the yard. Sammy crossed two fingers on his left hand and began talking without facing her. "Who. . .?" He licked his lips and paused. "Why did you come to see me the other night?"

She rocked gently in her chair and looked forward. Even as she spoke, she made no eye contact with him. "Why do you ask?" she said in a dry voice barely above a whisper.

He ignored her question. "How friendly are you with Dellwood?"

She screwed up her face and paused for a moment. "Business. We are business associates. Why do. . . ?"

Sammy interrupted her and raised his voice as he turned to look at her. "Is part of your business together knowing all about my personal life? 'I just happened to be at Emory right near your apartment,'" he said, mimicking her German accent. He made a scornful face and continued in his faux German. " 'I'm so sorry to hear about you and your wife.'"

Rosvita, still facing the yard, began to breathe audibly, and Sammy noticed that her hands shook. *I was right*, he thought. *She would tell me to get the hell out of here if I wasn't.*

He stood, went to the railing on the deck and leaned against it. "You see, I went to Mo's house to ask him a few questions related to Dellwood. He was all smiles at first, but as soon as I started to get down to the nitty gritty, he starts looking like he's just been told he has only a week to live. Lo and behold, the next thing I know, you show up at my apartment like Mata Hari." He got off the railing and walked in front of her. She slowly raised her head and stared at him.

"I began to ask myself some questions, like how much do I believe in coincidence? Then tonight I discovered this." He unzipped the front pocket of his anorak and took out the recording device. Rosvita was bug-eyed, but her face remained expressionless. Sammy thrust the device within inches of her nose.

"What is this thing you are showing me?" she whispered.

Sammy held it in front of her, but her hands, still shaking, remained on her lap.

"It's a recording device—the kind you attach to some poor sucker's phone when you're trying to . . ." He turned the recorder on and played a few seconds of his conversation with Siggie. "To spy on someone!" he yelled.

Rosvita put her head in her hands and began to sob. Sammy figured he had her against the wall, and now was the time to apply the pressure. "When I came downstairs from fixing a drink, there you were, pretending to be looking over my family albums, crying like you are now." Again he mimicked her accent: " 'I'm so sorry this happened to your family, I feel so ashamed,' blah, blah, blah. That's when you must've planted the device."

She looked up at him and, with tears streaming from her reddened eyes, shook her head.

"What did that asshole Dellwood ask you to do?" Sammy was standing over her now and yelling at her, "Mesmerize me, sleep with me, anything to find out what I knew, and maybe, just maybe, try to convince me to keep my mouth shut?"

She raised her head, glared at him, then stood and walked to the sliding glass door. She took another look back at him, then opened the door and went inside.

"I want some answers," Sammy yelled. "Don't walk away from me like I'm some kind of figment of your goddamn imagination." He followed her inside. "You know what the hell's going on, and I'm not leaving here until you talk."

She had her back to him, and all he could see was her body vibrating from head to toe. She seemed to be convulsing while standing up. With her back still facing Sammy, she wiped her face with her gray sweatshirt.

"Please sit," she whispered as she turned to face him. "We have much, very much to talk about." She pointed to the love seat near Sammy and said, "Please."

"No," he shot back. "I want answers now."

She continued to cry for several seconds then pointed to the seat. "Please," she whispered, "please do sit. You will need to sit for what I must tell you." She wiped her eyes and pointed to the seat at the same time.

Sammy took a deep breath and sat. Rosvita sat next to him on the love seat.

While looking down at her hands, she spoke deliberately. "I have wanted to tell you, especially after I found out for sure." She raised her head. "But I promised myself I would not, that it would be wrong to do so after all these years."

Sammy slammed his hand on the coffee table in front of them. "What the hell's going on here? What is all this cryptic shit?"

She stared at him. "Remember I told you I lost my parents during the war?"

Wary, he nodded.

"And that I lived in an orphanage for a few years, before being adopted by a couple from a village on Lake Constance—Freidrichshafen?"

"Yeah, yeah. Sure," Sammy said. "But what the. . .?"

"Well, all that is true, but I never told you about my *real* parents. I was four when they died, so I have some memory of them. My mother, who was probably quite young when I was born, was very beautiful. We lived with my maternal grandmother in what was then Upper Silesia. The name of the village was Rybnik—it is now in Poland." She closed her eyes for a moment and then continued. "We had a nice little stone house in the forest. My grandmother always told me how fortunate we were that my father was an officer of the German army, so we were never hungry—despite the war, food arrived every week or so."

Sammy stirred. "Okaaaay . . . But what does this. . . ?"

She put her shaking hand in the air to stop him, then wiped her eyes with her sweatshirt and continued. "We seldom saw my father. I was told he was so important that Hitler could spare him only for short periods. When he did come home, he would arrive in an open car that had two flags on the front. It was like a knight returning to his castle. He was a very tall, handsome man." She stopped for a second, shook her head and took a deep breath. "He wore a beautiful uniform with polished black boots, and the shiny medals and insignias on his chest sparkled in the sunlight."

"Holy shit! Is there any point to this story?" Sammy asked in a subdued tone. He moved to the other end of the love seat. "I mean, everyone's seen the old black-and-white movies with the Germans and their Iron Crosses, open cars, and all that crap. If your real old man was a Nazi big shot, tell me now and quit all the bullshit. I mean, you didn't pick your parents. It was an accident of birth. Plus the fact, I didn't come over here for any damn history lesson. If it helps, on behalf of the entire Jewish population, we forgive you, Rosvita. Okay? Now, what the hell has any of this got to do with you bugging my apartment?"

Rosvita ignored his question and continued. "I was young, but I remember that my father paid a lot more attention to Grandmother than he did to Mommy. I mean, he kissed Grandmother more and whispered things that would make her smile. She was very pretty and young herself—maybe not more than forty.

"One night I heard sounds from Grandmother's room. It sounded like someone was hurt; there was groaning. I opened my door and saw Daddy coming out of Grandmother's room with no clothes on. He went directly into my mother's room."

Sammy threw his arms in the air then slapped them down on his knees. "I ask you again, Rosvita: Is there a point to this story? The big German official was dipping his wick in two places. So what? I want some answers, and I want them now." He stood, took a step toward the glass door and slammed his hand against it. "All I've been getting from everyone lately is a bunch of maybe this and maybe that and all kinds of other veiled bullshit."

"Maybe we should take a walk, get some air," she said.

"Yeah, great. Why not?" he answered humorlessly, shaking his head.

Rosvita put on a green mackintosh, which she zipped halfway. They walked out the front door and headed toward the park. It was a cool night and a light mist fell on them as they walked up the hill on Eppington Road and onto the foot and bike path that circled Chastain Park. Both walked with their hands in their pockets.

She cut a look at Sammy, then stared straight ahead. "I didn't understand what was going on, but I knew Daddy loved Mommy, because in the spring of 1944, she told me I was going to have a baby brother or sister. I was very excited.

"The baby was born in January of 1945," Rosvita went on. "Unlike so many people in those days, Mommy had plenty of food while she was pregnant, so my brother was healthy and beautiful, like my mother and father. But, Daddy didn't come home when the baby was born. No food came either. We were forced to search the woods for nuts, berries, and roots. Mommy and Grandmother promised me Daddy would come soon and everything would be okay—there would plenty of food."

Sammy zipped up his anorak.

"One day, Mommy and Grandmother were sitting by the wood stove in our house. I was in the bedroom, but I could see them and overhear their conversation. Mommy got up, baby in her arms, and paced in front of the fire, telling Grandmother what she'd heard in the village. As she talked, Grandmother shook her head and had a look of disbelief on her face. Finally, Grandmother began to cry and put her face in her hands."

Sammy looked over at her as they walked, hoping he could see from her face what this was all about, but she had a blank look that gave no clue.

"Mommy was saying that my father's army was losing the war and he might be punished. A few months after my brother was born, Daddy finally did come home. He looked terrible. Instead of his beautiful uniform with all its shiny buttons and medals, he was wearing striped rags that smelled terrible. That night, he went into Grandmother's room without even speaking to Mommy and me. I don't think he even looked at his son."

Rosvita didn't speak as they passed the Horseradish Grill, where a number of people were dining and having drinks under a canopy. She began again when they were out of earshot of the restaurant.

"The next day, while playing in the woods, I heard loud noises coming from our road. We rarely had visitors, so I ran to see who it was. When I reached the clearing near the house, I saw a bunch of men—soldiers—going in the front door. They were not like my father's army—their uniforms were strange. I sneaked around the back of the house for a better look. The window was too high, so I stood on the wood box."

She reached in her coat to retrieve a tissue, then began to wipe her eyes. It took her a full minute to regain her composure. Sammy was silent.

"May we sit for a moment?" she asked.

He figured he'd heard this much of her story, so why not let her get to the big finish?

They sat on the low stone wall that ran around the park. "I didn't understand what I saw. Grandmother wasn't dressed, and some of the soldiers took turns lying on her. There was a little man dressed in the same terrible uniform Daddy had come home in. Near this little man was a tiny, scraggly woman wearing similar rags. One of the soldiers pushed the little couple toward a closet. Then he gave the man a gun. The man looked at it and handed it back, but the soldier was determined. He handed it back to the little man, but again, the man shook his head—over and over he shook his head. They went into the closet. I could not see, so I moved my crate. When I stood on the crate this time, I saw my father, his hands behind his back, hanging on a rack in the closet. The head soldier grabbed the gun from the little man, walked over to Grandmother, and shot her in the head. He went to Father in the closet, shot him, then cut him open with a knife."

"Jesus," Sammy said, now calmer. *If this were a true story, good God, Rosvita has witnessed some ugly scenes.* "Who were—?"

She interrupted his question. "I fell to the ground. I figured Mommy and my brother would be next. I moved into the woods near the side of the house where I hid in a gully. The soldiers were leaving. I was praying that Mommy was hiding in the cellar with the baby—maybe she heard the trucks and was able to get down there. Suddenly, Mommy was dragged from the house. It was very cold, and I remember she had on only a little flowered dress. They asked her some questions, then forced her back into the house screaming. Then, moments later—maybe it was longer, I don't know—I heard shots and the soldiers came out of the house with big smiles on their faces."

Sammy peered at her. "Who were these guys, Gestapo? I mean, did your dad piss them off by trying to surrender to the allies or something?"

She didn't look directly at Sammy but stared toward the street. "I was so scared, I was wet with sweat and freezing cold at the same time. My hair was matted, and my clothes stuck to me like I'd had them on for weeks, but I was safe in the woods for the time being." She looked at Sammy. "The officer, he was a Russian. That's who all the soldiers were. He took the two little people dressed in rags to the truck. Then suddenly another soldier ran from the house. In his arms was my baby brother. My mother must have hidden him in the grain cellar, which was empty. The soldier threw my brother onto the snow and waited for instructions. The major leaned out the truck's window and did this." Rosvita passed her index finger across her throat.

Sammy felt his own throat.

"The soldier pointed a gun at my brother. I closed my eyes, but there were no shots. When I looked up, the frail, ragged woman was lying in the snow on top of my brother, protecting him. She was screaming something in a language that was very much like German. She kept saying it over and over and over again." Rosvita covered her hands in her face and sobbed. Seconds later, tears streaming down her face, she raised up her head, peered at Sammy and said, "I will never forget what she was yelling at that soldier: '*Mare kinder nicht! Bitte, Nachum, sorgt ihm, mare kinder nicht.*' I later learned that it wasn't German . . . it was Yiddish, and the woman was pleading for my baby brother's life."

Sammy stared at Rosvita, his chest barely able to contain his pounding heart. He felt light headed, so he got off the wall and sat in the grass behind it. He put his head between his legs, trying to keep from fainting. *There was no way she could know that phrase—the one he'd heard so many times in the middle of the night.*

Rosvita knelt down beside him and began to stroke his hair. She spoke softly. "The officer laughed and then called the man's name and said the name of a place. Then, a while later, it may have been only a few minutes, I don't know . . ." She broke off into sobs.

He looked at her, his mouth wide open, his breathing audible. Rosvita regained her composure.

"The soldiers left. I stayed in the gully for a long time. The little woman continued to lie on top of my brother, covering his body with hers. She picked him up in her arms and began to sing a haunting song in a language that was not Yiddish, but was different from anything I had ever heard. I do not know the words, but the tune was a beautiful one." She hummed the melody he knew so well, and he heard the words in his head: *Henai matov uma n'ayim shevat achim gam yachad.*

Sammy said nothing.

She wiped her eyes, then sat next to him and put her arm inside his, looking at him as she spoke. "Eventually, she and the man picked up my brother and carried him down the road. I wanted to scream, but I thought maybe there were more soldiers, so I stayed in the gully and watched them take my brother away from me forever." She stared at the ground. "I have carried with me the words the Russian soldier said to the two little people who saved my brother's life. One was a name, a Jewish name—the Russian called the little man a Jewish name. The other was the name of a place. Do you want to know what those were?"

Sammy nodded.

"As the trucks drove away, the Russian soldier laughed and yelled at the little man and woman. He said, 'Nachum Zychilinsky, you go to Treviso! I don't give a damn.' I *have* never and *will* never forget those names."

Sammy jumped up and glared down at Rosvita. He opened his mouth to speak, but nothing would come out. His eyes—crazed and frightened—asked the question his mouth could not. He stood above her, staring at her face.

"Sammy, you were born in Upper Silesia in January, 1945. Your given name was Gottfried Heydrich. Your natural father, Rudolf Franz Heydrich, was the Gestapo chief of Auschwitz-Birkenau." She rose and faced him. "He was responsible for deciding who would live and who would die, who would be part of medical experiments and who would be shot for target practice. My—*our* mother and grandmother—" She looked into Sammy's face and peered into his eyes. "They were his wartime lovers."

Fighting off tears, he yelled, "You made all this up! You got me to tell you that my parents were Europeans, then looked at all our old pictures and then . . . you and Dellwood made the whole goddamn thing up so I wouldn't . . . " He ripped off his coat and threw it on the ground. He gave the coat one fierce kick after another.

"Why the fu—" To his horror, he realized he was beginning to shake all over and couldn't stop. "You *are* guilty just like I thought," he yelled. "The jig's up! Ol' Sammy's gonna spill the beans and send a few worthless pieces of shit to the can. So, Rosvita, the conniving German bitch decides she'd better come up with something to save her ass, and boy did she come up with a doozy.

"Okay, so you got the Yiddish saying right, the one about the children. Hell, a lot of camp survivors probably said that. Big deal. Or maybe you bugged my parents' place, too?" He picked up his coat again, and this time he threw it at her.

The coat stuck to her for a moment then fell to the ground. She spoke coldly and with resolution. "Whether you like it or not, Sammy, my original name was Anna Heydrich, and I am your sister."

Sammy finally surrendered to the truth, fell to his knees, and began to cry. She knelt down and held him.

CHAPTER TWELVE 12

ROSVITA HELD HIM IN HER ARMS, and he didn't resist. They sat on the ground, huddled together for several minutes. When he'd calmed down, she helped him up, and without speaking they walked across the street to the Horseradish Grill. It was bustling, but they found a booth and settled in.

"Rosvita," Sammy said, folding his hands on the table. "You know I've got to check this out with my parents. How are you so sure about all this?"

They ordered a glass of wine and some focaccia. When the waiter left, Rosvita spoke. "After I was adopted by the Schulers, I told my new parents about my brother." She smiled and continued, "So they set out to find this Nachum Zychilinsky and see just what he and the little woman had done with my brother. Fortunately, the Nazis, they were compulsive record keepers, so we were able to establish that such a man was in Auschwitz and that, to the best of everyone's knowledge, he had survived that place. My adopted father, who from this point on I will just call my father, had some contacts after the war with the Joint Distribution Committee and found that a Nachum Zychilinsky left Venice with a wife and a child in the winter of 1947."

"Yeah, but there may've been twenty Nachum Zychilinskys at Auschwitz," Sammy said. "I mean, the name, it's probably like, uh, David Stein in the U.S."

Rosvita shook her head. "I know, I know, but this man and his family left on a ship from Venice headed to Palestine in the winter of 1947. Do you know what city is near Venice? Treviso. Venice is its port."

Sammy thought for a second. "There may've been other Nachum Zychilinskys in Treviso."

She nodded and shrugged her shoulders. "Maybe. Anyway, the family boarded a ship in Venice, the *Joshua Wedgewood*, but that ship never made it to Palestine. We could not find them and assumed that if they eventually made it to Palestine they might have changed their names to Hebrew ones—you know, like Ben-Gurion did. By 1954, we had exhausted all our sources of information. We had no idea what happened to the family."

She reached across the table for Sammy's hands, but he slid them into his pockets. "There's too much confusion," he whispered, looking at her.

She nodded. "For many years, it stayed that way until something very strange and wonderful happened. While I was finishing my engineering degree, I worked weekends as an aide in the trauma unit at the Grossharden Clinic in Munich. Our unit was chosen to treat the most severe Israeli casualties of the Six-Day War. The German government had offered transportation and medical care—an inexpensive act of good will since there weren't that many severe injuries. This is when I met Shalom Esrov, an Israeli officer and American expatriate." She smiled when she mentioned his name.

"Despite a terrible wound that required removal of most of his colon, he remained strangely upbeat and positive. I would visit him on the weekend because he was nice and I knew he liked my company. Every Saturday and Sunday, I would sit with him and listen to his stories.

"I asked Shalom why he had gone to Israel. He told me that after the experiences he'd had, it was the only place in the world where he could live. He was not even born Jewish, although he had converted by the time I met him. He had been in the American Merchant Marine during World War II and after the war. He tried various jobs, but nothing was as satisfying to him as the sea. He was only twenty-three then, so the idea of punching a time clock wasn't for him. Anyway, he was hanging around the Brooklyn Navy Yard looking for work when he heard about a job that sounded exciting and exotic—taking European refugees, survivors of the Nazis, to Palestine. He signed up as a boson on the *Joshua Wedgewood."* She paused. "The *Wedgewood,"* she repeated, leaning toward Sammy. "Can you imagine how excited I was?"

He remained motionless and did not reply.

"Shalom told me that the ship sailed to Biarritz, France, then down the Iberian coast through the Straits of Gibraltar. There, the British Navy became its constant companion. He said that the British would come alongside the ship and ask their destination. The radio operator of the *Wedgewood* played 'The Chattanooga Choo-Choo' every time the British asked. That was it. No answer, just the music. The British followed the ship around Sicily, into the Adriatic and all the way to Venice, where the *Wedgewood* docked for two months while the ship was refitted for passengers."

"Must be when we got on," Sammy muttered to himself.

"What?" she asked.

He shook his head.

All around them, waiters and busboys cleared tables and put out fresh tablecloths, and there was the hum of conversation, but Rosvita and Sammy appeared to be in a cocoon and didn't notice.

"Shalom, then known by his given name, Donny Estes, told me that in late March of 1947, the crew was put on alert. They were to sail within the next forty-eight hours, so they boarded the ship and waited. Two days later, at about eight o'clock in the evening, the crew heard singing coming from the shore. The voices got louder and louder and had a haunting quality, almost like the sounds came from the heavens, and angels were serenading the men. The sailors looked through the evening mist, and soon they saw a mass of people—women, toddlers in arms, children holding hands, men. Some walked, some hobbled on makeshift crutches, and some were carried." She paused and took a deep breath. "All were singing a beautiful song that none of the crew had ever heard.

"It was *Hatikvah*—the song of hope that was to become the national anthem of Israel. Shalom taught me the words:

> *As long as there's a Jewish soul that vibrates at the*
>   *pit of the heart,*
>
> *And as long as our eyes turn toward the East seeking Zion,*
>
> *As long as our tears flow and the Jordan waters Tiberias,*
>
> *And the Wall waits for us,*
>
> *Only with the last of the Jews*
>
> *Will the last hope disappear . . ."*

Sammy closed his eyes and covered them with his hands. His body shook with sobs. Rosvita wiped her eyes on a handkerchief. "These poor, desperate people, given up as human refuse by most of the world, were singing . . . singing a song of hope. Children who had been treated like cattle all their lives—singing."

The waiter brought the wine and bread. He asked if they wanted more, but neither of them said anything, so he left.

Rosvita continued. "Shalom told me he realized then God had chosen him to perform a sacred task. These poor, hopeless people had to get to Palestine. The ship arrived in the port city of Varna, Bulgaria, on the Black Sea, where she picked up another load of survivors. It was here, in Varna, they changed her name for the final trip back through the Dardanelles, across the Aegean and on to Palestine. People on the ship covered the name *Joshua Wedgewood* with a Hebrew name. I'm not sure how you say it—something like, *Nishoma Yisroel*, The Soul of Israel."

Sammy shook his head. "Oh, Rosvita . . . oh, God, oh, God!" He nestled his head in his hands. "That's it—the ship—the one we were on. We have the pictures." He tried to wipe his forehead with a napkin, but his hands shook too much.

She helped him with the napkin, then spoke. "Twenty-five miles off the coast of Palestine, they sighted land—the snow-capped top of Mount Carmel. Shalom said there was more joy and celebration than he had ever seen. People were singing and dancing the hora; round and round they went in a circle, singing at the top of their lungs. Old men dressed in black robes and top hats rocked back and forth in prayer. Men, women, and children climbed up on the rail and the mast for their first sight of Palestine. The ship listed as everyone scrambled to catch a glimpse of the shore.

"About ten miles off the coast, they saw a British destroyer. A voice from the British ship announced over a megaphone, 'You are now entering territorial waters. If you resist, the blood will be on your head.' The *Nishoma* began to turn south to avoid the ship when the destroyer began heading straight for them at full speed.

"Soldiers in helmets and gas masks, carrying clubs and rifles, were standing on the destroyer's deck. Suddenly, the destroyer rammed the *Nishoma*, and a platform extending eight to ten feet was lowered from the destroyer onto the ship. Soldiers poured over the platform and used clubs, high-pressure hoses and tear gas to subdue unarmed, defenseless people. The British imprisoned the passengers on a ship fitted with barbed wire." Rosvita sighed. "These people knew all about barbed wire. The *Nishoma* was towed to port. Some jumped overboard and swam to shore. Most of the refugees were sent to a Displaced Persons camp on Cyprus called Zylotambou."

"Sh—that's, that's how they, uh, we ended up in Cyprus," Sammy whispered. "How'd you figure out . . . I mean, what made . . . makes you think I'm who you think I am?"

"We, my parents and I, tried to find out what happened to the family. We had a few leads here and there but finally gave up. No one seemed to know where you and your family had gone.

"Then, years later, in the early eighties, I was at a wedding of my friend's cousin in London. I started talking to this man from Brussels—deNeuwe was his name, but that is of no consequence—and after awhile, he tells me that he is a big shot in an organization that researches war criminals. I was not too interested in him, but every time I turned around at the wedding, he was there. I was about to tell him to get lost, particularly since he was getting drunker all the time, when he tells me he also runs a business helping refugees locate their families—for a nice fee, of course. I think he was trying to impress me with his brains or his money. I don't know which.

"It took him eight months and a lot of my money, but one day deNeuwe calls me and tells me that Zychilinsky became Lansky and that the family was now in a town outside of Atlanta, Georgia, named Cordele. I called a friend of mine from Munich, who was working for Siemens in Atlanta. My friend travels all over the Southeast taking care of Siemens X-ray equipment. He knows that I am looking for my brother, so I say to him that maybe if he is in this Cordele he could snoop around and see what he can find out. He goes to your . . ." She hesitated for second. "He goes to your parents' store, and there right in the front window, he sees a newspaper article which has been—how you call it," she thumped her head for second, "the wax . . ."

"Laminated," he said.

"That's right. Anyway, this article is from the local paper, and it says with great pride that Samuel Lansky, M.D. is now practicing urology in Atlanta. So, I knew where you were at last."

Sammy was quiet and seemed to be in deep thought. "How'd you get here? I mean, you in Atlanta, me in Atlanta—too strange."

She nodded. "We didn't meet by accident. I couldn't just fly to America, present myself at your door and say, 'Here I am: your long, lost sister, who you never knew you had.' I told you I worked for MAN as an engineer. Along the way, I got a graduate business degree, so after I found out where you were, I started to look for German companies that had offices in this part of the U.S. and who needed someone with my skills. When I learned that Dornier had formed a medical division and that it's North American headquarters would be here in Atlanta, I applied and got the job."

He closed his eyes and leaned forward, his head resting on his hands. He spoke softly. "If what you've told me is true, I was born *before* the end of the war in 1945. I've spent my whole life thinking I was born in 1946 in Treviso. My whole life—not to mention my birth—has been a lie." He leaned across the table and whispered with clenched teeth. "A damn lie."

The waiter came by and asked if they wanted anything else. Both of them looked at their untouched wine and focaccia and said no. He handed them the check, which Sammy paid. They wandered out of the noisy restaurant without either of them hearing a thing. It had begun to mist more densely, so she zipped her coat all the way up and he pulled the hood over his head.

"After the night I met you at the party, I went home and stood at the mirror. I took off my makeup and pulled my hair back." She looked at him as they walked back to her house. "There you were, staring back at me. I decided that I wanted to make absolutely sure you were my brother, so I came to your apartment, and when I saw the pictures and you told me what your parents' real names were—I knew I had found you after almost forty years of searching."

It began to rain. "I had decided that it would be wrong to parachute into your life, but I knew my life would not be complete if I did nothing." She stopped, took his arm, then brought him to her and hugged him. "You gave me no choice." She looked up at him. "I didn't come to Atlanta to work for Dornier or Dole or anyone else—I came here to see, maybe meet, my brother."

He held her. "I'm so confused. I don't even know who I am," he said.

She backed away from him and, as the rain pelted them, she spoke in a stern voice. "You are not like anyone else, Sammy. You can never be like anyone else. Your life was saved by Frieda and Nathan in more than a physical sense. You carry the genes of a psychopathic murderer, as do I. Yet your parents' love overcame that, as did mine." Frieda and Nathan are inside you as if they blew life into you. You have their spirit, their soul—their *nishoma*."

CHAPTER THIRTEEN 13

HE LEFT ROSVITA'S HOUSE AROUND 9:30 P.M., and there was no doubt about where he was going. There were perfectly good reasons not to make the three-hour drive to Cordele: By the time he would arrive, his parents would have been in bed for hours, and their side of the story wouldn't change before morning. Plus the mess with Dellwood was still hanging over his head, and he needed his own sleep to think straight about solutions to that problem. But Sammy went anyway. The next time he stood in front of the mirror to shave, he wanted to know whose face he was shaving.

Except for the rhythm of the windshield wipers, the drive to Cordele was completely silent. Just Sammy and his thoughts. After he got south of Macon, there was no one else on the road. He drove past flat expanses of darkened farm land as he had done many, many times before. This time he felt like he was in the twilight zone. *How could his parents hide the circumstances of his birth? On the other hand, how could they tell him? Apparently, Rosvita had made peace with her demons; could he? Could he trust Rosvita? Sister or not, she was in pretty heavily with her company and, by extension, Dellwood. What was her deal with Dellwood? Lover? Friend? Accomplice? Who planted the recorder at his apartment?*

He arrived at his parent's house, turned his car lights off, and drove slowly into the driveway. He could hear the crackle of the gravel under his tires and felt his car bump as he drove along the uneven path. Sammy had thought about calling his parents, but he'd known that doing so would only give them three hours of extra worry, so he hadn't. After closing his car door with great care, he turned toward the house and immediately saw the blinds in the front window part slightly. He took a step toward the door, and within seconds, the outside lights came on and his mother came rushing out.

"Darling, what is the matter? What is this with the coming home in the middle of the night?"

"Schmuel! You're home!" screamed Nathan, bolting out the door as if shot from a cannon.

"Nachum," Frieda said, hitting her forehead. "The whole neighborhood, they are asleep. You don't have to broadcast it." She wagged her finger at her husband. "That voice of yours, the way it carries, oiy."

Sammy hugged both of his parents, placed his arms around their shoulders and led them toward the house. "Let's go inside. I've got to talk to y'all about something."

"This is the middle of the week, not the weekend. *Vos tut zich?*" Nathan said as they went inside.

"I'll, uh, I'll explain."

They sat in the kitchen. Frieda, a pained look on her face, began to cut some coffee cake, but Sammy asked her to sit.

"It's Rachel, she is sick," Frieda said, trying to cut the cake. Her hands were shaking so much, she finally put the knife down and walked over to the table.

He helped his mother with her chair, then stared at his parents for several seconds. The only sound was the creak and whir of the fan. He took his mother's right hand into his, placed it on his cheek, then brought it to his lips, and kissed it. He did the same with his father. He looked at one then the other and whispered, "I love you." Tears filled his mother's eyes.

"I just, uh . . . I just . . . met a woman." He stopped for a second and looked down at the table. "I didn't just meet her, but, that's, uh, not really important. Anyway, I just talked to a German woman. She says . . ." He let out a long breath. "She claims to be my sister."

Sammy closed his eyes when he saw his parents turn toward each other, pause, then hold hands.

"Who is this woman, Sammy?" asked Frieda in a soft voice. Tears streaked her cheeks.

"Her name is Rosvita Schuler. She says she was at the little house in Upper Silesia when I was . . ." Sammy struggled to speak as his voice cracked. "When I was saved by you."

Nathan turned away from his wife and peered at Sammy. "This woman, what was she doing there at the little house?"

It is true, thought Sammy.

"She was hiding in the woods. She saw the soldiers rape and kill her grandmother, kill her father . . . they heard a baby cry . . . the soldiers pulled a young girl out of a cellar, then a baby. The soldiers killed the young girl. The baby was saved when a half-dead woman, a survivor from one of the camps, fell . . . the woman fell on the baby and pleaded for his life. Rosvita saw the whole thing. She says I'm that baby—her brother. She says my father, the one who was killed . . ." Sammy closed his eyes and hesitated for a moment. "She said he was Rudolf Franz Heydrich, Gestapo chief at Auschwitz."

The silence was deafening. Frieda cupped her hands and looked down at them. Tears fell from her face onto the table. She spoke softly. "I had not seen an infant since 1942. There were no babies in the Lodz ghetto and, of course, none in Auschwitz—they were murdered as soon as they got off the transports." She looked at Sammy and wiped her eyes. "I had not talked to God for two years.

When I saw you lying there in the snow, I began to talk to Him again." She shook her head and continued.

"We carried you in our arms and on our backs for days, weeks, months—through Slovakia, then northwest Hungary along the River Raha and finally into Slovenia. Everywhere there were people walking: faceless, hopeless people. The war was over. There were no planes, no tanks; just chaos, hunger, death—it was the end of the world.

"You got sick, very sick, outside of Postoina in Slovenia," Frieda continued. "We stayed there for three months—October until December of 1945. There was a hospital in Ljubljana, but to them we were garbage, so they would not help us. We told a priest in Postoina who you really were. He saw that you were not circumcised—maybe we were telling the truth. He gave us shelter in the monastery and food and what medicine there was. We only had to make one promise—one promise."

Nathan had been staring at Frieda. He turned toward his son and, in a voice choked with emotion, he spoke. "The priest made us promise to leave you there to be raised by the monks. We made such a promise to get the medicine you needed. We made friends with a local dairy farmer who delivered milk to the monastery. When the time came to leave, he agreed to take you away in secret. We stuffed your bed to make it look like you were asleep, then we hid you in the farmer's cart. We left hurriedly on foot and met him several kilometers outside of town."

Nathan looked down at his hands and rubbed them, then he continued. "We were walking with you down an old road when a man driving a hay wagon stopped. He asked us who we were. We made up some story, but he knew we were Jews. He told us there were many robbers and such on the road. He said . . ." Nathan hesitated and glanced at Frieda. She nodded and he continued, "He said that he had seen enough killing and misery, that we could hide in his hay if we wanted to. Down the road, the wagon, it stopped again. We were buried under the hay, but we could hear someone asking about 'two filthy Jews and a Christian baby.' The wagon driver said nothing and was told to move on."

Nathan extended his hands toward his son's. "Sammy, there were many good Christians in Europe—the milkman and the farmer were only two."

"This is very true," said Frieda. "The mayor of a little Italian village gave us a ride across the border into Italy in the trunk of his car, then we walked to Treviso. There were lots of people there in Treviso. They were flying the flag of *Eretz Yisroel* and learning how to handle weapons and that sort of thing from members of the Hagana. It was very exciting."

Nathan, tears streaming down his cheeks, looked at Frieda and said in Yiddish, *"Es iz geven zaier gut."* She pinched his cheek, then leaned over to kiss him. "One day," Nathan said as he turned toward his son, "one of the Hagana leaders—his name was Dov, Dov Sharon—he came to us and told us we would need papers to enter Palestine. He told us we could put anything we wanted on those papers since we were going to begin a new life."

Frieda interrupted Nathan. "We put our names down as Nachum and Fruma Zychilinsky and your name down as Schmuel Zychilinsky—this even though we . . ." She paused and looked at Nathan. "Even though we were not yet married and you were not . . .

"As he was walking away, Dov turned to look at us and said, 'I assume Schmuel was born in Treviso in, let's see, January 1946? It will be easier. Fewer questions.' Well, it was only April 1946, but we weren't going anywhere soon, so Nathan and I shook our heads okay. Then, with a smile on his face, Dov asked us a question. 'Do you know Moishe Safra?' I nodded and he continued. 'He can help you. He is a mohel.' "

A smile crossed Nathan's face as he spoke. "We took you to a small creek and used it as a *mikva*—you know *mikva*, don't you, Sammy?"

Sammy nodded recognition of the ritual bath.

"Anyway," Nathan said, "we used it to convert you. It wasn't in Eretz as we hoped, but we made do. Mama and I were married on board a ship bound for Palestine—the *Joshua Wedgewood*, which became the *Nishoma Yisroel*."

Sammy tried to hold in his tears. As an adult, he had never cried in front of his parents, but now his effort was futile.

"We told you about Cyprus," said Nathan, rubbing Sammy's hands. "We stayed less than a year. Mama and I wanted to go to Palestine very badly. Our desire never weakened despite the endless waiting for a visa."

"You were never well on Cyprus, Sammy," Frieda broke in. "You coughed, spit up, had constant diarrhea, and slept fitfully. Papa and I feared you would die. When the Atlanta Jewish Federation offered to take in refugees, we signed up. We came to this country in November of 1947, as Nathan and Frieda Lansky, with our son, Sammy. At the end of that month, the United Nations voted for partition, but we still would not have been allowed to go to Pales—Israel, because independence was not declared until the British left in May of 1948."

Sammy looked at his parents with reddened eyes. "Everything she said was true."

"This woman?" Frieda asked.

Sammy nodded.

"We," Frieda said, motioning to include Nathan, "have never known of her existence, but yes, everything she told you is true."

Sammy cleared his throat. "Mama, Papa, I owe everything good in my life to you."

"We love you, our darling."

Sammy stayed in Cordele the next day. He walked around his old haunts but didn't call any of his friends. He needed time to think about what he had just learned. He did call Rosvita in Atlanta—*My sister*, he thought as he dialed the phone—to let her know what he'd found and to apologize to her for his behavior.

"I did what I had to do," she said. " I will never know if it was the right thing or not."

"Yeah," he said quietly

"I love you, my brother," she whispered into the phone.

He put the receiver in the cradle and wept.

◆ ◆ ◆

SAMMY RETURNED TO ATLANTA THURSDAY. He called Mary, told her he had the flu and wouldn't be in for a day or so. Maybe, he would stay out until Monday to make sure he got better.

He sat in the hall of mirrors and stared at the hollow pits that housed the once-bright-green eyes of the son of Rudolf Franz Heydrich. He did not shave, shower, nor change clothes the entire time. The only conversations he had were with himself, and his sole sustenance came from the dark, peaty liquid which lay in a bottle that never left his side. There were no days and nights, just minutes in a continuum filled with his attempts to figure out the past.

At first the drink made him mellow and, in his heart, he thanked Frieda and Nathan for all their goodness and love. His eyes filled with tears as he thought about how much they must have loved him to let him find his own way in life after they had sacrificed so much for him. He thought about calling them and telling them, but he didn't. He picked up the phone ten times to call Rachel just to talk to her, but he couldn't bring himself to do it.

As more of the clear glass of the bottle appeared, Sammy began to curse everything and everyone. After all, his real father had never wanted him, the Jews in Cordele and Fitzgerald had avoided him, Sylvia and Mo thought he was a joke, and the one woman he loved had told him he was a loser—a rainbow missing a few colors.

Why was I born in the first place? he asked himself. *Here I've been trying to wedge a Jewish boy's heart and soul into this goddamn carcass of mine. No wonder I haven't been able to get it right. I've lived the Great American Dream, and that's all it's been—a dream. There isn't one thing about it that's real. I'm nobody, nothing, not even a statistic . . . unless lies are statistics. After all, I don't even really know my name. But, what's a name anyway, huh? A silly moniker chosen out of a book, history or who knows, maybe thin air? Who gives a damn, right?*

He shuffled in his chair, and the legs screeched against the hardwood floor. He leaned forward so he would not miss one word he was saying to himself. He was a foot from the mirrored wall now.

His eyes reminded him of the time long ago when he was in Canada on an engineering job. A friend had suggested a walk along a crater near the little town of Kamloops. It was dusk, the edge of the crater black from lava eons old. As they got to the top, they could see a sliver of glacial green water in the depths, a lake made millions of years ago, but fading out of sight for the night. Now, in the hall of mirrors, he could see a sliver of green peeking out from the black hole that his eyes had become.

At least now it all made sense to him—his mother's screams in the middle of the night about the children: "No more children, Nachum, no more children. Tell him no more children," she would wail in Yiddish. Yes, now it all made sense to him.

He put his face against the mirrored wall and smelled his alcohol-drenched breath.

I've pursued happiness, he thought as he fell out of his chair and slumped to the floor, *but it could never be mine.* He looked at the floor and was unable to raise his head. The patterns in the wood made him dizzy. *It could never be mine because I am no one! Nobody!* He put his hands against the mirrored walls and yelled, "Nothing!"

When his brain cells had had enough, he passed out on the floor. It went on like this, day and night, for the rest of the week and on into the weekend. Each morning, his head was in a vise and his gut burned, but he didn't care.

◆ ◆ ◆

SUNDAY AFTERNOON. SAMMY, CLAD IN WORN OUT SCRUBS that stuck to his body, lay sprawled on his belly in bed, his right leg touching the floor to keep the room from becoming a carousel, a round spot of drool on the sheets where his head rested. *Bang! Bang!* Sammy wondered why his landlord had to pick today, of all days, to work on the outside of his apartment. *Bang! Bang! Bang!*

He lifted himself into a sitting position, felt a wave of nausea, and fell back onto the bed. *Bang! Bang! Bang!* With his right foot firmly anchored, Sammy pushed himself up, then managed to roll off the bed onto the floor. Holding onto the side of the bed, he got to his knees where he stayed for a minute. *Bang! Bang! Bang!* Slowly and wobbly, like a fawn's first steps, he rose and struggled from the bedroom. *Goddammit, why the hell does he have to play Mr. Fix-It on the weekend?* he thought.

Sammy went to the kitchen for water as the banging continued. Glass in hand, he started to negotiate the steps. *If he doesn't stop, I'll go to a damn hotel.* Two steps down, Sammy halted when he heard, "Sammy! Sammy! Open up, please." It was Rosvita. She was banging on the door. He took a big gulp of water and poured the rest on his head.

"Wait a minute, wait a minute," he said. His mouth was full of cotton. He put the glass on an end table and opened the door.

"Oh, no, you look terrible," Rosvita said, scrunching her face.

Sammy grabbed the door for security. "You have a keen insight into the obvious." He bent over with his hands on his knees, then sat on the floor. Rosvita helped him to a couch and closed the door. She sat in a small wing chair near his head.

"Where have you been? I have been calling and beating on your door since Friday. Your car was here. Your office said you were sick."

Sammy stretched out on the couch and stared at the ceiling. "You ever see those horror movies where the people are trapped in an elevator and the sides of the elevator are closing in on them?"

Rosvita nodded.

He rolled over and looked at her. "Well, I'm the poor sucker in the elevator and the damn thing is about to press me like a shirt."

Rosvita leaned over and rubbed his matted hair. "What is going on?"

Sammy leaned up on his elbow and rolled his eyes toward her and sighed. "Other than the fact that my whole life has been an illusion, my wife left me cause I'm worthless, my real father used babies like skeet, and I would've been in the Hitler Youth had things worked out a little better for the Nazis, everything is perfect, just perfect. Oh, and lest we forget, Dellwood has me pegged as his whipping boy. Life is just grand." He fell back on the couch and stared at the ceiling.

Rosvita slid her chair toward the middle of the couch. She cleared her throat and spoke in a near whisper. "What is this between you and Dellwood?"

Sammy rolled his eyes toward her, but said nothing.

Rosvita took his hand and held in hers. "Friday morning, my boss said Dellwood was worried about you—about your loyalty."

He bolted up then fell slowly back into a supine position. "My loyalty? To what? What the hell is he talking about?"

"Loyalty to your partnership, loyalty to the other doctors in the state."

Sammy spoke as he pulled himself into a sitting position. "Tell me, Rosvita, why would Dellwood tell your boss anything? Your boss's job is to sell and service lithotriptors, plain and simple. Why should he give a shit about anything Dole or I do?"

Rosvita clasped her hands together and looked at Sammy. "Our company makes the only lithotriptor in the world, and we are selling them all over the world, but the truth is that when it comes to profitability, the United States is the oak tree and the rest of the world is the acorn. This is the largest free market health care system in the world, and we are poised to make billions of dollars. In most countries, there are but a few machines, all in major cities. In the U.S., there will be more machines in some states than in entire countries, including many in Europe. Mind you, Sammy, the profit on selling the machine is a healthy one, but it pales in comparison to the money made selling the individual electrodes for the machines and servicing the machine."

Sammy shook his head. "So? What's that got to do with me and Dole?"

Rosvita hesitated for a second. "Dole told my boss you are spying on Dornier and feeding information to the insurance companies and hospitals. He claims you are trying to stir up bad publicity about things like how much money we are making because you are involved with a competing lithotriptor that is in the works. An American company called MedStone."

"What the fuck? That's a pile of crap. In the first place, I've never heard of this MedStone. In the second place, what kind of info could I be feeding anybody about anything that they don't already know?"

Rosvita continued. "Dellwood also told my boss that you . . ." She hesitated again. "He said that you might be involved in something illegal, something to do with stealing money from the doctors in your partnership."

Sammy threw a pillow across the room. "Fuck that bullshit. If anybody's doing anything illegal, it ain't me. It's that asshole, Dole. In fact, in the next few days, I may be able to—" He stopped midsentence and looked at Rosvita.

"Why did your boss tell you all of this? Does he know, you know, about us?"

She shook her head. "No one knows who didn't know before except, of course, you and your . . . your parents in Cordele. He told me because I am VP of North American sales and because Dellwood has his ear."

Sammy leaned over, arms on knees, head down. He spoke through clenched teeth. "Dellwood is a lying bastard and I intend to prove it."

Rosvita rose and went to the small window across from Sammy's couch. Looking out the window, with her back to Sammy, she said, "Be careful, Dellwood is dangerous. I have seen him in action."

"I'm shaking in my damn boots."

She turned toward him. "He is vicious. He is the puppeteer, and everyone in his sphere are puppets. If he can't control you, he tries to destroy you."

"I'll wrap his goddamn puppet strings around his neck and choke the little sonofabitch."

She took a deep breath, moved deliberately across the room and sat next to Sammy. "When my boss told me Dellwood was suspicious of you, it was not the first time I had heard this accusation. I would have said something, but there has been no time since—since we—you—found out about us."

"What do you mean?"

"When I first came to America, Dellwood tried everything he could to get me in bed. I guess you have noticed his attraction to taller women. I resisted, politely at first, then not so politely. He told me how important he was to Dornier and that he could have me sent back to Munich if I wasn't 'nice' to him." She smiled sardonically. "He said this was the way business got done in the U.S., and if I didn't like it, he promised to make life miserable for me."

"Shhh—what a bastard," Sammy said in a low voice.

"Finally, he realized my pants were permanently off-limits to him, so he tried another strategy. A few months ago, we were sitting in a bar in Florida after a meeting. He says we will be good friends and no hard feelings if I will do one thing for him. While he is talking to me, all I can think about is how to get this weasel out of my life. Then he says there is this young doctor who is causing problems, disrupting things, and he wants me to become friends with this doctor and see what is going on."

Sammy and Rosvita stared at each other.

"I am just about to tell him to crawl back under his rock, when he says the young doctor is you. He wants me to spy on my own brother."

Sammy leaned back on the couch. "Son of a bitch. That's why you were at the Gordons' party. The whole time I figured you were his date. Did he ask you to bug my apartment? Was it you who put the recorder here."

"No. I have no idea about that. You must believe me."

Sammy shook his head. "I do. I'm sure they have their ways."

He sighed. "I'll be damned. Dellwood's been setting me up as a fall guy just in case."

Rosvita had a pained expression. "In case of what?"

Sammy's shook his head back and forth. "In case I found out what he and Henry had done. How they set this whole thing up to steal money from the doctors—lots of money. They must've figured I wasn't quite as comfortable with things as they wanted me to be."

Rosvita's eyes filled her face. "Are you—are you sure of these things?"

He shook his head. "No, not at all. But, I am awful suspicious."

She took Sammy's hand. "Be careful. Dellwood is dangerous. Very dangerous."

"So am I," he said. "So am I."

CHAPTER FOURTEEN 14

SAMMY RETURNED TO WORK MONDAY. He was no longer scared. He was pissed off. Dudley Kessler's secretary called him first thing Monday morning to make a dinner appointment for Thursday, but gave him no hint as to what the lawyer had been able to find out.

As he was dictating in between patients on Thursday, Sammy heard Mary on the intercom. "Dr. Lansky, Mr. Dolt is on the phone."

"Hello," Sammy answered.

"Sam! How are you! The board needs to meet. Tonight, 7:30 at Mo's. Okay by you?"

"Well, I have an appointment . . ." As usual, Dellwood had left him speaking to himself, the only response being the sound of the dial tone on the other end.

He immediately called Kessler's office and tried to reschedule but was told that Kessler would be out of town until late Thursday afternoon. Sammy furiously rapped the desk with his fingers. *He's the puppeteer, and those in his sphere are the puppets.*

That evening, he stopped by the apartment on the way to Mo's. He went to his closet and took out a billy club Buddy had given him years before when he moved to Atlanta to attend Georgia Tech. Along with the strange gift had come an hour of detailed instruction. Sammy put it in the back part of his belt, putting his sport coat on to conceal the weapon. As he walked to his car, he wished Buddy were with him now.

♦ ♦ ♦

When Sammy arrived at Mo's, there were three cars in the driveway. He recognized Dellwood's Rolls and Henry's Audi, but not the third one. Getting out of his car, he peered into the Gordons' garage and saw their three luxury autos. He checked his billy club one last time then rang the doorbell. Mo's kid, who was wearing paraphernalia from five different sports teams, greeted him with: "They're upstairs in his office."

"Thanks," Sammy said, patting the kid on his New York Yankees hat.

"Sam! How good to see you!" Dellwood threw his arms wide open as Sammy entered. "Isn't it wonderful to see Sam?" he said, turning to Henry.

Henry rose and shook Sammy's hand. Mo stood behind Henry and took Sammy's hand next. Sammy noticed two men helping themselves at the bar.

"Let me present two friends, Sam," Dellwood said, guiding Sammy toward the bar to introduce the men. "This is Jake Monas, and this is Jules Steele." They shook hands, and Dellwood invited everyone to sit.

Mo started for his desk, but Dellwood got there first and settled into his huge leather chair. Henry selected an upholstered chair with an ottoman and, without comment, Mo sat down in its companion. The leather couch was available, but the two newcomers chose to stand. Sammy sized up the situation as Buddy had taught him: *Make sure your hands are free, stand if possible, never get on lower ground, never allow anyone to be at your back.* As he stood against the fireplace facing everyone, he could feel the billy club.

Monas, his thick, black hair glued in place with mousse, made eye contact with no one. He was about thirty-five with a medium build and a chronic tic made up of several parts: his right eye closed, then his right cheek twitched, and he finished with a bizarre twisting of his head which made him seem more like an owl than a man.

Steele was different. About six-two, he had tidy, curly black hair. His beady, dark eyes were locked on Dellwood. Both he and his companion bought their suits high-end retail: superfine wool with broad pinstripes, two-tone shirts, French cuffs, collar pins, and Hermès ties.

"I want to start this meeting of the board of directors of Georgia Stone Institute by offering an apology to one of our members." Dellwood leaned back in Mo's chair. "After all, it *was* Sam Lansky who told us about this cash cow we call lithotripsy. Yet, inadvertently," Dellwood said and cupped his hands together, "we failed to explain the business in its entirety to him. Please accept our collective apology, Sam." Dellwood leaned forward and smiled at Sammy.

Sammy looked at Mo, who stared at Dellwood to avoid eye contact.

"Apology for what? You guys have been apologizing for days, and you still haven't said for what," Sammy said in a loud voice. *Be loud, and it will make you bold.* Buddy's countrified instructions continued to play in his head.

Dellwood got up and sat on Mo's desk. He slithered around on the desk until he was perched on the front edge of it, then he crossed his legs.

"The doctors own Lithotripsy Associates, which was established so that some guy from, let's say, Cordele, or any other godforsaken outpost in Georgia, could send his patients to Atlanta and not have to come here himself. Lithotripsy Associates also guaranteed that its members would share in the Georgia Stone

Institute's profits generated by the technical charge for the machine. Are you following me so far?"

Sammy nodded. "Go on," he mumbled.

Dellwood adjusted his paisley ascot and began to parade in front of the desk. "And," he said with great theatrics, "*share* they do. We," he said, pointing to Henry and Mo then Sammy, "agreed to be oh, so generous and allow the docs to have twenty percent of the profits—the board gets eighty percent." Dellwood shrugged his shoulders. "Fair, if you ask me. After all, we set the whole thing up, didn't we?" Dellwood looked at Steele, who shook his head.

"The docs paid for it," Sammy said in a loud voice.

Dole smiled. "But, we," he emphasized, pausing to open his arms, "own it. Within a year, we'll have similar arrangements in Florida, Tennessee, North Carolina, South Carolina, and Virginia. We stand to make over five million bucks per board member per year."

Dellwood returned to the edge of the desk, sat, and folded his arms across his chest. "Everything was going great. We were on our way to millions. Then one of us started asking questions—something about two different checks. Right, Mo?" Dellwood turned to his right to look at Mo.

"Uh, yeah," Mo said, looking straight at Dellwood.

Dellwood got off the desk, walked over to Sammy and patted him on the shoulder. "*Well*, I said to myself, *Dellwood, that's your fault.* Yeah," he said, shaking his head. "I said to myself, *You never explained things to Sam. How could you expect him to understand?* So that's why we're here, my dear boy. That's what this meeting's about—to explain *everything* to you since you seem to have an insatiable need to know." Sammy looked down at the shorter man. They were face to face.

"This setup is all perfectly, one hundred percent legal. The docs are making money and have no way of knowing they're getting screwed. Doctors are so busy they never have time to look into all the minute details of a deal; that's why they make so many lousy investments. This deal is a win-win—they win, we win. Do you know the only way this could get messed up?"

Sammy could feel the shorter man's spit hit him in the face, and he could smell liquor on Dellwood's breath. Dellwood stood on his toes and spoke in Sammy's ear. Sammy started to move but decided to play the game. "A loud-mouthed, stupid asshole," Dellwood said in a loud whisper, "who refuses to be a team player. That's the only thing that could mess this up."

In a fit of pique, Dellwood grabbed Sammy's collar with both hands, then let go. He paused for a moment to calm himself. "That's right, this is a golden goose unless someone too stupid to wipe their own ass messes it up. The docs are happy now, but all they need is one person—one single, solitary, itsy-bitsy, insignificant, moronic person—to tell them what's going on, and all of a sudden things could start to unravel."

He adjusted his sport coat and backed away from Sammy. "I mean, when I hear my name mentioned in the same breath as the word *criminal*—" Dellwood paused for a second and used his handkerchief to wipe his face. "I get very uneasy. Very uneasy. You, Sam, don't want me to be uneasy, do you?"

Sammy stood his ground. He could feel the presence of Dellwood's two large "friends" and kept them in his peripheral vision, just as Buddy had taught him.

Dellwood had the floor, so he continued. "You didn't think we'd quit when you found our little recording device, did you now, Sam? We've been recording your conversations at the office and home for some time now. We know about Siggie and Kessler, and what your wife or ex or whatever she is, thinks about all of this."

He paused, turned, and looked across the room at Monas and Steele, then at Mo.

"When I hired you," Mo said in a quiet voice, and without looking at Sammy, "I thought you loved money as much as we do. I thought you were one of us." He looked up, and with a pained expression on his face, glanced at Sammy. "Now, I feel like I let a traitor into our camp." Mo lowered his eyes and shook his head.

Sammy, now completely on his own, stared at Mo, unsure how to react.

Dellwood slithered over to Mo, put a hand on his shoulder, and squeezed. He wore a plastic, sorrowful look on his face and spoke with pithy sarcasm that oozed from his mouth like thick goo. "It's my fault, Mo. My fault." He continued to pat Mo on the shoulder and shake his head.

"Sam, how do you suppose we got the license for lithotripsy for the whole state of Georgia, huh? Do you think I won over the licensing people with my good looks?" He put his hand behind his head and cut a pose. The two men at the bar laughed, though they didn't smile.

"How do you suppose we worked it out, so to speak, to have a monopoly over lithotripsy for the next five years? Think about it, Sam," Dellwood paused. "Not another lithotriptor in this whole damn state for five wonderful years." He stared at Sammy for a second, then a sickening smile creased his face. "Bet you didn't know that, did you? Anyway, after five years, the technology will have changed, the machines will be mobile, and there'll be one on every . . . single . . . corner. But it won't make a damn bit of difference to us, and you know why, little Sam?" Dellwood opened his arms and shrugged his shoulders.

"Because we'll be so rich, we won't give a shit. The state of Georgia has given us the right to print money for the next five years. Which brings me back to my original question. How'd we get all this, Sam? Ever wonder?" He paused for a second. "You can't possibly believe the state just gave the machine to us, not when Emory had all those nice credentials." He glared at Sammy for a moment with an air of deadly seriousness about him. "They gave it to us, my dear Sam, because we gave them—*money.*"

Dellwood put his hand in his pocket and pulled several one-hundred-dollar bills out of a fat wad stuffed into a gold money clip. With a laugh, he threw them at Sammy. Monas joined in with a raspy, staccato grunt that sounded like a machine gun. When Sammy stared at Dellwood, the laughter stopped.

Dellwood flicked some lint off his burgundy linen coat, pranced past Henry and Mo, stopping in front of Monas and Steele.

"We've got four members of the state health planning board on our payroll—been that way for years. We've never had any trouble getting anything we want. We also make healthy contributions to five state representatives, including the Honorable Thomas McFie, Speaker of the House. They get what they want—big bucks. We get what we want. Am I making myself clear?" Dellwood raised his voice and stared at Sammy.

Sammy said nothing. He could feel sweat running down his back, pooling at his belt line.

Dellwood got right in Sammy's face again, spitting with every word. "This deal is foolproof—it has layer upon layer of insulation—all you had to do was accept your checks and shut up." He grabbed Sammy's collar and, again, pulled it tightly around his neck. "How could I expect to make a businessman out of some backwoods redneck who grew up swallowing gnats and had parents who could hardly speak English? No wonder you're a loser,

Lansky—you were born a loser." Dellwood let go of Sammy's collar and began to affect a laugh that made him double over.

Sammy stood at the fireplace, looking at Dole. Buddy was talking to him again: *Never let an advance go unchallenged—bullies are always shocked when you fight back*. He grabbed Dellwood by the coat with his left hand and slapped him hard with his open right hand. Before anyone could react, Sammy brought his hand back, striking the right side of Dellwood's face with his fist and knocking him to the floor.

Monas and Steele lunged for Sammy, but backed up when Sammy flung open his coat, whipped out the billy club and swung it at them. Monas fell back, tripping over Dellwood, who was still on the floor. Sammy grabbed Dellwood's head, spit in his face, and let go. Mo and Henry sat wide-eyed and motionless.

Steele, his composure regained, drew a knife, crouched, and crept toward his prey. Sammy grabbed the wrought-iron poker from the fireplace and thrust it toward his attacker.

"I'll shove this right up your ass if you take one more step," he yelled at the man. "You, too," he said to his partner, who had gotten to his feet. With his jaw clenched and an animalistic mask on his face, Sammy glared down at Dellwood, then surveyed the room with his eyes. "And . . ." He looked from one man to another. "I'll beat this cocksucker to death." Another Buddyism: *Get meaner and further down in the sewer than your opponent.*

Steele backed off but held the knife in plain view.

Sammy raised the poker. Dellwood drew himself into a ball and covered his head as the poker cut through the air, stopping inches from his skull. Sammy stepped over the shaking Dellwood, pushed his thugs aside and started toward the door when he heard a voice speaking behind him. It was Dellwood's.

"We all know whose idea this was, Sam," Dellwood said. "You talked us into it, set up the whole scheme. If you tell anyone about this, you're the one who'll end up in jail. It's three against one, you bastard."

Sammy turned around and saw Henry trying to help Dellwood to his feet. Dellwood yelled as he got up, "Maxwell Cherry's got all the bank records." Dole grabbed Henry by the arm then continued in a loud voice, "Turns out that Sam Lansky stole millions from the urologists in the state and his dear friends, his business partners. Can you believe it? Did all of that without anyone knowing about it." He let go of Henry and walked toward Mo. "Can you believe that our dear, trusted friend, Sam, your partner, stole from you?"

Mo shook his head without looking up.

Henry whispered, "Terrible, just terrible."

Dellwood stood behind Mo's desk. "We," Dellwood said, pointing to Henry and Mo, "didn't know anything about it." He started to laugh uncontrollably. "No telling what an investigation will turn up. You're going to go to jail till you're an old man, Lansky. You'll be eating mush off a tin plate while Henry, Mo, and I will be dining with our banker in Zurich."

He hit his chest as he began to laugh. "I'm so smart I scare myself."

Sammy stood in the doorway facing Dellwood, listening to his ranting. He had the billy club in his right hand.

Dellwood continued to laugh so hard he had to wipe his eyes with his handkerchief. "We've got such pull, you'll go to jail for so long you'll forget what life on the outside is like."

When Dellwood had finished, Sammy pointed a finger at him and said with a smile, "You've made a big mistake, a big mistake." He looked around the room, stopping for a second at Mo, who turned from Sammy's gaze. "All of you," he said, turning to include

Mo, "have made a big mistake." He then rushed down the hallway and out of the house.

"That son of a bitch is gonna be trouble," said Monas.

Dellwood, who had stopped laughing, turned to Henry and said, "Time to put Plan B into action."

◆ ◆ ◆

SAMMY WAS SCARED AS HELL, but Buddy had been right. He had stared danger in the face, had not backed down, and he felt a strong rush. He shifted his Saab into overdrive as he hit I-285, looked behind, and didn't recognize any of the cars that had been at Mo's. Just as he hit the turnoff for I-75 south, he bolted up in his seat when he heard a beeping noise. *Whew, just the end of the tape!* He reached in his jockey shorts and took out a small tape recorder. He pushed rewind, then listened as Dellwood put himself, Henry and Mo right in harm's way. He removed the cassette and slipped it into his pocket.

Sammy wasn't going back to the apartment. They would expect him to do that and could nab him easily. There was only one place he could go and be guaranteed of his safety even if followed. He had enough gas to get there. No reason to call, because where he was going, there was no phone.

He got off I-75 at exit 33. As far as he could tell, no one had followed him. He drove down Rock Top Road to the turnoff and proceeded slowly toward the cabin. It was after eleven, and illumination from the full moon cast an eerie glow on the road like low-wattage outdoor lighting. As he approached the clearing, a thick cover of trees blocked the light from the sky, and the road twisted like an S. No one would go this way at night without headlights. Buddy wanted to know when he had visitors.

Damn, Sammy thought. *I hope the crazy son of a bitch has all of his marbles properly aligned. Otherwise, I'd be better off with the enemy.* Sammy got out of his car, leaving his headlights on. He walked toward the cabin; no lights were on. *Where were the dogs?* he thought.

"Buddy," he called, "it's me, Sammy, I need your help." He bounded up the steps and tried to look in, but the shades were drawn. He knocked, then banged on the door. No answer. He looked around the back of the house. Buddy's truck was there, but all he heard was the intermittent pop and buzz of a bug zapper. *Shit,* thought Sammy. *Where the hell is he?* As he walked back to his car, Sammy heard the unmistakable sound of a shotgun cocking. He looked back but saw nothing.

"It's me, Buddy—Sammy, Sammy Lansky," he yelled. "Where the hell are you? Come out, please. I need your help." Sammy looked around. His throat was dry, and he could hardly speak. "C'mon, Buddy, please."

From the darkness somewhere in the woods, Sammy heard a raspy voice, "What's your Hebrew name, and what's mine?"

"I'm Schmuel, you're uh . . . you're, um, Bezalel."

Suddenly there were lights everywhere. Sammy shielded his eyes with his hands. When he had adjusted to the light, he looked around. Buddy was ten feet from him, shotgun in hand. There was a pack of at least ten mangy dogs within five feet of Sammy, waiting for Buddy's command.

"Damn. Good thing I remembered your name," Sammy said, taking a deep breath and bending over.

"What you doin' here?" Buddy asked with a blank look on his face.

"I need a place to hide for a few days." Sammy wiped his forehead.

"What you done?"

"Nothing . . . nothing, nothing." Sammy leaned over. Without speaking, Buddy grabbed him by the arm and helped him onto the small porch, which led into a combination den/kitchen and dining room. The only bedroom and bathroom were in the back of the cabin. Buddy had no phone or air conditioning, but he did have indoor plumbing. He helped Sammy onto a rough-hewn couch and got him a glass of water.

"Thanks," Sammy said as he lay down.

Buddy nodded.

Sammy looked around, surprised to see that the place was spotless. There were no dishes scattered around, and no clothes laying on chairs.

"What kinda trouble you in?" Buddy asked.

Sammy told Buddy about the night's events, trying not to get too technical when it came to the money.

"These here greaseballs, one of 'em got slicked-back, black hair, and he's so nervous, looks like his head gonna fall off?" Buddy asked.

Sammy raised his eyebrows and looked at Buddy. "You know them?"

"Naw, but I seen 'em."

"Where?"

"They been around the store for the past coupla days."

Sammy wiped his face with his shirt again. Buddy had all the windows open, but even with a fan on, it was hot and sticky. Every few seconds, he could hear the bug zapper.

"What the hell for?" Sammy asked. "Why've they been at the store?"

"That's what I been tryin' to find out. They done showed up on Tuesday, walked around the store, bought a few things here and there, then left. But they ain't really left. They been 'cross the street at Cindy's."

"What the fuck? They're one step ahead of me," Sammy uttered under his breath.

Buddy looked at him curiously but asked nothing about the last remark. "They been following Mama and Papa home, then goin' down to the ho-tel for the night."

"You see them today?" Sammy asked.

"They was here till afternoon, then they was gone."

"Oh, shit," mumbled Sammy.

"Don't worry none, Sammy."

"What do you mean?"

"I set me up a bivouac in Mama and Papa's backyard soon as I saw them greaseballs follow 'em home."

"You mean you're camping out in my parents' yard?"

"Not exactly, not where nobody can see me. I'm using that old fort Edbo Towns built for you boys."

The Lanskys had three quarters of an acre behind their house. Years before, Edbo Towns, Clete's dad, had built a first-class treehouse, removable steps and all, near the property line. Sammy and his friends, who had been studying ancient Egypt in school, had formed a club named the Sphinx Society. The treehouse was its headquarters. Sammy built a Heath Kit radio, and the club members would sit in the treehouse on Saturdays and listen to Al Ciraldo and Jack Hurst do the play-by-play of the Georgia Tech football games. When it rained, the gang would gather for Mama's cookies, lemonade, and a game of Monopoly. But that part of the property had become so overgrown with kudzu, Sammy hadn't paid any attention to it in years.

"How'd you even find that old place?" Sammy asked, taking a sip of water.

"Hell, it ain't moved. Anyway, I got me a command post all set up. Mama and Papa cain't see me, but I'll know if anyone gets near the house."

Sammy looked at Buddy. "How's that?"

"Got me some walkie-talkies from Radio Shack over on Seventh. Got me one at the front and one at the back of the house. Got me one of each up in the treehouse, too. I got 'em marked front and back, so I can know where the perpetrator's comin' from. I'd be there tonight if I hadn't followed them boys outta town earlier."

Sammy looked down and whispered, "Umm, I know where they went. What the hell have I gotten myself into?" He turned to Buddy. "I think you should start sleeping over there every night. The bad actors I've gotten involved with in Atlanta apparently hired these boys to scare me. Seems like they're thinking about putting the squeeze on Mama and Papa to try to get me to cooperate. I can't think of any other reason those boys would be here."

Buddy gave Sammy a look that made him a little uncomfortable. "Anybody lay a hand on Mama and Papa will D I E." His eyes took on a demonic look. "By the strength of these hands," he said, showing his paws to Sammy, "they will die."

Sammy nodded. "I don't know for sure, but they may be trying to convince me to keep my mouth shut about some stuff they've pulled."

Buddy stared at Sammy. "What exactly you done, Sammy? You ain't done nothing illegal, have ya?"

Sammy shook his head. "Hell, no." He paused and looked at the floor. "It's so complicated, I'm not even sure I understand half of it. But I got something here," Sammy confided, reaching into his pocket and pulling out the tape, "that'll put them under the jail. It's a confession."

"Hmm," Buddy said, looking at the tape.

Sammy motioned for Buddy to sit. "Listen, I need for you to go over to Perkins Hardware in the morning. Go to the red and white UPS box. It's outside next to the post office boxes. I want you to get me a mailing envelope out of that box—it's called an overnight letter. It's a cardboard envelope, about yay big," he said, demonstrating to Buddy. "Red and white. Got that?"

Buddy nodded.

"Also, I'll need something to write a note on. Got any paper?" Sammy asked.

Buddy nodded.

"Good. Tomorrow, I'll send this tape to an attorney in Atlanta. Things ought to be okay after he listens to it." Sammy put the tape back in his pocket. "Where's the nearest pay phone? One where I won't be seen?"

"Bar down on Rock Top 'bout a mile. Ain't nobody there in the mornin'."

"Good, I'll go down there first thing tomorrow and make a call," Sammy said, thinking he needed to let Siggie know what had happened.

"Want me to tell Mama and Papa anything?" Buddy asked.

"No, definitely not," Sammy said, shaking his head. "They'd want to go to the police, and I think we'd better keep everything quiet until I can get in touch with this lawyer."

After Buddy went to bed, Sammy lay on the couch, unable to sleep. *Monas and Steele had been here scouting the place. Dole is dangerous, as Rosvita had said. If I don't cooperate with them, they may harm my parents.* He sat up, his heart racing, sweat pouring down his face and torso. *I'm their prisoner, and they've got Mama and Papa as hostages. Who knows? Maybe they've got the D.A. on their payroll, too. Shit, they've got me by the short hairs. Any time—for who knows how long—I get out of line and threaten them, they can . . .*

He fell back on the sofa and stared, wide-eyed, at the wooden beams above him, unable to believe that, without the slightest intention, he might be responsible for completing the work of his natural father. Hauptsturmfuehrer Rudolf Franz Heydrich, baton in hand, pistol at his side, the double dagger of the *Schutzstaffel* on his cap, had tried to kill Fruma and Nachum. They had survived that endless night and had taken him—Gottfried Heydrich—from certain death to a rich life in another place with another name. Now, Gottfried Heydrich was no more, and Sammy Lansky was going to have to risk *everything* to protect them.

CHAPTER FIFTEEN 15

Buddy had worked out the logistics. He would park his car at the Crisp County Tourist Office after work, sneak back along Seventh Avenue to Sixth, climb the vine-laden fence on the Lansky's property line, and ascend to the treehouse. He had fitted a finely woven netting over the front of the structure to protect himself from the bugs and kept a sleeping bag, canteen, some granola bars, and a flashlight in a plastic storage box near the back of the platform.

There had been no sign of the store-watchers since Thursday morning, and Sammy was still at Buddy's place, not saying much. After Mama and Papa closed the store on Saturday night about eight, Buddy drove to the tourist office, started to park, then decided he'd better drive past the house to make a quick check for unwanted cars. He circled the block twice, saw nothing unusual, and went back to the tourist office.

After leaving his car, he maneuvered his way through the strangling kudzu to the Lanskys' fence. He climbed into the treehouse, donned camouflage pants, a black shirt, and a camouflage vest. He lit a citronella candle, screened its light, then crawled back to his storage box and took out a pair of night-vision binoculars he had ordered years ago from *Soldier of Fortune* magazine. He saw nothing unusual, and there was no sound from the monitors, so he spread out the sleeping bag, lay down, closed his eyes, and listened to thousands of crickets talking to each other.

A piercing noise cracked from the back monitor. He jumped up, reached for the binoculars, and scanned the house but saw nothing. Jamming the binoculars into his belt case, he picked up a knapsack with a sawed-off baseball bat strapped to it, put his hands and feet on the outside of the ladder, and slid down. He moved silently around the periphery of the yard. When he got within a few feet of the carport, he hid behind a huge rhododendron. He waited for a moment, and when he saw and heard nothing, he crawled into the carport. Nothing seemed amiss. He removed the bat and put the knapsack on his back. *Probably just a cat or coon*, he thought. *Better check it out.*

He went to the back door and found the screen open. Gently he nudged the door—it was ajar. Someone had gotten into the house without his knowing it. Buddy took his hunting knife out of the pack, put it onto his belt, and held the bat with both hands as he pushed the door open and tiptoed into the dark and quiet kitchen. He could hear the familiar sound of the attic fan as he crept past the living room and the den. He heard something—muffled sounds—coming from down the hall. He moved deliberately, whispering to himself, *Mama, Papa, where are you?*

At the top of the stairs to the basement, he stopped abruptly. He could hear someone yelling from below.

"You tell that dumb shit son of yours to keep his fucking mouth shut, and you'll never see us again. If he squawks, you folks are gonna die. We're never gonna be far away."

Buddy went down one step at a time, pausing when the voices paused. He looked between the wooden slats along the stairway and could see a stocking-covered head moving violently as it spoke. "Yeah, if he's quiet, you live. He talks, you die. It's that simple. Oh, by the way," said the man, twisting his head even farther right, "nobody, especially these redneck police down here, can protect you from us. We're everywhere, and if your son doesn't behave himself, we'll be your worst nightmare."

Buddy got to the bottom step and saw Nathan and Frieda, bound and gagged, on their knees facing two men, both of whom had stockings on their heads. Nathan had blood streaming from his forehead into his eyes. Frieda's dress was torn from the shoulder to her breast. Her eyes widened when she saw Buddy behind the attackers. Steele followed her gaze, but he was too late. Buddy's bat hit the right side of his face with such power that his cheekbone became one with the side of his nose as the force of the blow hurled him against the concrete wall of the basement. Buddy moved toward Frieda and Nathan, but Frieda's eyes cut left, telling him of danger. He followed her look and saw Monas staring at him with a gun. Their eyes met and were locked on each other for a second. Buddy swung his bat at Monas' face, and as Monas saw the wood flying at him, he fired. The bullet crashed into the upper part of Buddy's right chest, below the collarbone, just as his bat smashed into the enemy's face. Buddy felt no pain, only a deep, searing sensation. He took the end of his bat, beat Monas unconscious, clubbed Steele two more times, then freed the Lanskys and hugged them. Breathing heavily, Buddy picked Frieda and Nathan up, and ascended the stairs into their bedroom.

"What is going on? Who were those men? How did you know to come?" Frieda asked as rapidly as she could form the words.

Buddy helped them get out of their bloody clothes and, after he had them settled down on the bed, went to the bathroom to retrieve some supplies, returning with iodine and small towels.

Nathan spoke. "Bud Dee . . ." Buddy signaled for him to be quiet while he tended to the wounds.

"Bud Dee." Nathan pushed the large man's hand away from his face. "We should call the police. We *must* call the police right now." Nathan's speech was impaired slightly by a swollen lip. "These men, they are serious, they mean business, and we have to call right away. If not the police, then at least Dr. Hattaway. He should look at these wounds, no?" Nathan rose and took a step toward the phone. Buddy gently pushed him back on the side of the bed.

"Look, Sammy may be in some kinda trouble with these boys. Y'all don't know much about how the po-lice work, but some things is best straightened out before the cops ever know about it. This here may be a private matter that the law ain't got no business gettin' involved with. As far as your cuts go, you're gonna be okay without no doctor. Y'all best lay down here and let me take care of everything."

"But, we must—," said Frieda.

Buddy interrupted her. "Mama, Papa, y'all done taught me everything I know about bein' a good person. On Passover, after we been singing God's praise for six days, we only sing half of the prayer in His name the last day, on account of us feelin' sorry for all them E-gyptians what died when the Red Sea opened—them bein' human and all." Buddy put the supplies on the nightstand. "A lot of them E-gyptians was just doin' their duty, but some of 'em—like the boys what done this tonight—" He pointed to the Lansky's wounds. "They was so low down and nasty, they got what was comin' to 'em."

"But the police," Frieda said as she began to cry, "they will see that they broke in, they beat us. These men, they are dangerous men." She wiped her eyes. "The police need to take them to jail, have a trial. They know Sammy, they may have friends, they may try to harm him." She began to weep again and Nathan cradled her in his arms.

"We can't have anything happen to Schmuel," Nathan began, tears dripping down his face onto Frieda's head. "We have had enough taken from us already." He reached out and held Buddy's hand for several seconds. Buddy wiped a tear from his own eye.

"These boys ain't gonna bother no one around here again, 'specially not y'all and Sammy," Buddy said in a quivering voice.

Nathan sat on the edge of the bed, holding Frieda's hands in his. Buddy put his giant paws on top of theirs. After a few moments of silence, Buddy stood, pulled back the bedcovers, and helped the couple into bed. As he tucked Frieda under the covers, she lifted her head up and whispered into his ear, "Please don't let anything happen to Sammy."

Buddy held Frieda in his arms and whispered back, "Not while I'm alive, Mama."

He went into Sammy's bathroom and removed the towel he had stuffed under his black shirt. It was full of blood, but apparently Mama and Papa hadn't noticed because of his dark shirt and vest. His neck and upper chest were already quite swollen, and blood was beginning to dissect his right shoulder and cascade down his arm. There was a blast wound just below the collarbone where the bullet had entered. He took another towel and placed it under his shirt. Holding pressure with his left hand, Buddy walked slowly into the kitchen and picked up the phone. He opened the phone book, squinting as he got to the T's. He dialed the number, and on the fifth ring, a sleepy voice said, "Hello."

"Clete, this here is Buddy. You got to go get Sammy and get over here."

"Wha' the hell. . . ?" Clete said in a sleep-garbled voice. "You got any idea what time it is? What's going on?"

"Ain't got no time to explain. Sammy's over at my place. Get him. You boys come over to Mama and Papa's house. And don't waste no time doin' it."

Buddy hung up, took a deep breath, and walked into the basement again. Steele and Monas were groggy but waking up. Using his left hand, Buddy picked up Monas' gun and pointed it at them.

"Boys, you tried to hurt the only people what ever loved me. Now, you gonna have to pay."

◆ ◆ ◆

Forty-five minutes later, Officer Johnnie Underwood of the Cordele police passed by the Lanskys' house on his routine patrol. When he saw the lights, he glanced down at his watch. *Damn unlike the Lanskys to be up past midnight,* he said to himself, *much less two in the morning. Course, the store ain't open on Sundays, but still . . .* He drove around back, noticed the door was open, and went in. In the den, sitting by himself, chanting in a language Underwood had never heard, was Buddy Ambrose.

"What the hell's going on here, Buddy? Where're the Lanskys?"

Buddy looked up from his chanting. He stared at Underwood and the bulging of his eyes made the cop step back and instinctively reach for his gun. "Sleepin'. They're fine." Buddy spoke in a barely audible voice.

"What the hell're you doing here?" Underwood asked, looking around the room.

"Two boys broke in, I was passin' by, and I chased 'em outta here."

Underwood walked around the den, keeping his distance from Buddy. "They harm anybody, get anything?" he asked.

"Naw. I woulda got 'em, but they was two of 'em, so they got away."

Underwood stopped looking around and stared at the huge man, who swayed at the rhythm of his own voice.

"What these boys look like, Buddy?"

Buddy continued to rock. "Dunno. Had stockings on their heads."

"Well . . ." Underwood sat on the arm of a couch across from Buddy. "I mean, was they white, colored, tall, short?"

"White, real big, talked some language I ain't never heard."

"Shit, that ain't nothin' to go on," said the cop without taking his eyes off Buddy. "Was they speaking Spanish, Canadian, or what? How the hell am I gonna file a report?"

Buddy didn't answer. Underwood shook his head, looked around the room for a few seconds more, saw that nothing was disturbed, and left. He had no idea what had happened, but he had a pretty good notion that if someone had broken into the Lanskys' house and Buddy had caught them, they might not have gotten away.

The officer got in his car, opened his report book, held it open for a minute, then closed it. He could hang around and follow Buddy, see if he had the two boys. But, if Buddy did, odds were some lawyer from Atlanta would get them off on a technicality. No, he'd go back to the station and fill out a report saying the perpetrators had escaped. In the morning, when there were more deputies around, the Chief would want to launch a full-scale investigation. That was okay with him, but for now, he'd play a little solitaire and wait till the end of his shift.

❖ ❖ ❖

Underwood's taillights had barely disappeared when Clete's truck crept into the driveway. It was followed by another vehicle.

"Damn, I thought that cop would never leave," said Clete, jumping out of the truck and pulling his shotgun off the rack in the back. He opened the gun, checked for ammunition, and closed it.

Sammy hopped out of the other side. "Yeah, he might be back. Big Boy," Sammy said, looking at Big Boy Bates, who was getting out of another vehicle, "why don't you move the cars while Clete and I go inside, see what's up."

Big Boy closed his door and shook his head. "That cop ain't comin' back. Wouldn't have left if he was. Plus the fact, you boys might need me in there." He pointed to the house, then slapped his hip where he had a gun.

They agreed and slipped in the back door. Clete followed Sammy through the kitchen. "Awful damn quiet," he said.

In the den, they saw a hulking figure stretched out in a chair. "Buddy," Sammy whispered.

Buddy turned toward Sammy, and whispered, "Mama and Papa." He pointed toward their bedroom.

Sammy spoke softly to Clete and Big Boy. "You guys stay here with Buddy. I'll go see Mama and Papa." He ran into the Lansky's bedroom while his friends, weapons drawn, more cautiously entered the den.

When he flipped on a bedside light, Sammy found his parents half-asleep in each other's arms. Quietly, he sat on the side of the bed and visually examined their facial wounds. Frieda looked up at him with fuzzy eyes and started to scream, but she covered her mouth when she realized it was Sammy. She reached for him, and they hugged each other.

"Schmuel, Schmuel," she whispered, rocking back and forth with her son in her arms. "*Robonoy shel oylom*, God in heaven, you have saved my Schmuel."

Nathan's eyes opened. He wrapped his arms around his son's neck. "What is going on here?" Nathan asked.

"I'll tell you later," Sammy replied, holding his right hand in the air. "All that matters is that you're all right."

"And, Bud Dee?" asked Frieda.

"He's fine, fine. I just left him in the den." Sammy pointed in that direction.

"We are all right." Nathan said, sitting on the side of the bed. "You go thank Bud Dee, then you come back and tell us what is all this *tsores* we got here."

Sammy rose. "Just stay here, that's all I ask. I'll go talk to Buddy."

He kissed his parents, then went into the den. Clete had put his shotgun on the sofa and was kneeling at Buddy's side. Big Boy Bates stood over them, holding onto Buddy's chair. When Sammy entered the room, Clete's eyes met his. Sammy walked slowly over to Buddy, who was slumped down in the chair.

"Hey, Buddy, what happened?" Sammy asked. He popped Buddy on the shoulder, but got no response. Clete stared at Sammy nonstop.

Unable to remove his eyes from Clete's, Sammy sat down at Buddy's side and gently pulled the giant man's head toward him. When he did, he saw the massive swelling in Buddy's neck. He looked in Buddy's eyes and saw the vacant stare of death he'd seen so many times in the hospital. "Buddy, Buddy, it's me, Sammy." He shook Buddy, then suddenly smashed his fist against the huge man's chest. He began to pump on Buddy's chest. "Do mouth-to-mouth," he yelled at Clete. "Don't just stand there like a fucking moron."

Clete stared at Sammy and shook his head.

"C'mon Clete," Sammy said, his voice still raised, but now pleading instead of yelling. Again Clete shook his head. Sammy held Buddy's head in his hands and let out a scream that became a cry then a scream again. "Buddy! Oh, God, oh, God! No, no, no! Buddy!" He yelled the man's name over and over.

Nathan and Frieda rushed into the den when they heard Sammy's cry. They looked at their son—bent over and holding Buddy's head in his hand. Frieda threw her hands heavenward, fell to her knees and screamed God's name in Yiddish. Nathan fell upon his sons and began to sob and rock in prayer. Still on his knees and shaking uncontrollably, Sammy put Buddy's head down and faced his parents. They got next to him and were enveloped by his outstretched arms. "I killed him," he whispered. "I killed him."

◆ ◆ ◆

BUDDY HAD POINTED OUTSIDE AND SAID TWO WORDS to Clete and Big Boy before he died: "Revenge me." Big Boy left Clete to be with the Lansky family and walked around the property until he found Monas and Steele handcuffed to each other, their faces flush up against a large oak.

Big Boy stood above the two men. "Hmm, something here stinks," he said. In a moment, he realized what Buddy had done: poured Frieda's perfume all over them, enticing the gnats, mosquitoes, yellow jackets, and no-see-ums to infest the men's skin.

Big Boy looked down at the two men, whose faces were terribly disfigured, and shook his head. "You pukes gonna wish you'd stayed in the hole you come from. Messin' around in these parts was a major fuck-up."

CHAPTER SIXTEEN 16

MONDAY MORNING, CLETE AND RAYANN TOWNS drove Frieda, Nathan, and Sammy to the funeral in Fitzgerald. The Lanskys sat in the back of Rayann's Chevrolet station wagon holding hands and saying nothing.

Sammy had told his parents *a* truth, but not the *whole* truth about Monas and Steele and why they were in Cordele. He'd told them Buddy's killers had wanted him to get involved with some shady business and, when he refused, they had threatened him, causing him to seek Buddy's protection. Unable to find him, they'd tried to scare his parents. Sammy decided that, for now, the police should concentrate on finding Buddy's killers and not broaden their investigation.

"Sure was nice of Mrs. Kaminsky to have everybody over for the memorial lunch," Clete said, looking in his rearview mirror at Sammy and his parents.

Rayann touched Clete's shoulder and said in a soft voice. "It's called sitting shiva, honey."

Clete looked over at his wife and said in a whisper, "I knew that." He looked in the rearview mirror and directed his comments to the Lanskys. "I know y'all wanted to have the, uh, shiver at your house, but this here is more convenient—the church and the cemetery being down here in Fitzgerald and all."

"Synagogue," Rayann said, looking at him.

"What?" Clete asked, returning her stare. Realizing what he'd said, he quietly replied, "Oh, yeah, yeah."

They drove past the synagogue on Lee Street and out toward Evergreen Cemetery. Clete stopped in front of the blue-and-white arch, inscribed Fitzgerald Hebrew Congregation, and let the Lanskys out. There were already a number of people milling about the tent that had been set up in row T. Many of them waved fans in an attempt to circulate the steamy air. The cemetery had only a few skinny pines surrounding it, and they provided no shade. Sweat poured off Sammy's face as he guided his parents, one on each arm, toward the grave.

"Wait," Frieda said when they approached the Holocaust memorial. "I want to stop here for a second."

In the middle of the path was the granite and marble memorial the Kaminskys had given to the community. It was a large obelisk approximately twenty feet high, with a Mogen David (star of David) at the top. The inscription:

IN MEMORIAM

This monument is erected in memory of the six million Hebrew men, women, and children who met death at the cruel hand of the German Nazi government between the years 1933–1945.

Erected 1954

After they paused for a moment, Sammy escorted his parents to the family tent. Rabbi Phillip Kranz greeted them with condolences. Now the rabbi at Temple Sinai in Atlanta, he had been a student rabbi in Fitzgerald years before. The *chazzan*, who had taken a day off from teaching, was also at graveside. As a small crowd gathered, Sammy felt a tap on his shoulder.

He turned and saw Rachel. "How . . . how'd you know about Buddy?" he asked.

When she leaned over to speak, Sammy could see the glistening of perspiration and tears cascading down her face. "Mama called me. I'm so sorry, Sammy."

◆ ◆ ◆

BUDDY JOE AMBROSE WAS LAID TO REST in a plain pine box. As his remains were lowered into the ground, Rabbi Kranz recited the Twenty-Third Psalm, alternating English and Hebrew:

"*Adonoi ro-ey lo eczor.*"

"The Lord is my shepherd. I shall not want."

The *chazzan* sang the haunting *S'eem shalom*—grant peace. One by one, the few members of the congregation who were gathered shoveled dirt onto Buddy's coffin. Finally, Sammy and Nathan each took a shovel and put several mounds of dirt into the grave. As they worked, Rachel neared the family and sat next to Frieda. The older woman, tears streaming down her face, nestled her head under Rachel's chin and whispered in a scratchy voice, "This is the first member of my family I have ever buried." She wiped her eyes with a trembling hand, and Rachel hugged Frieda as they cried.

After Sammy and his father sat, Rabbi Kranz said, "Buddy Ambrose's body has left us forever, but as we stand here today to tell him goodbye, we know his soul, his *nishoma*, will now begin its journey to heaven." He turned to the Lanskys. "The family can say kaddish."

Sammy held one of his parents on each arm, closed his eyes, and listened as he heard them utter the ancient memorial prayer that had been said on too many occasions for too many people who had not gotten life's full measure. The only sound was a background chorus of sobbing accented by the murmurs of an ancient plea.

When the service was over, Rachel walked with the family to her parent's graves.

Ester Dziewinski
Born Lodz, Poland,
August 6, 1920
Died Fitzgerald, Georgia,
February 14, 1978

Avrum Dziewinski
Born Krakow, Poland,
January 5, 1916
Died Ocilla, Georgia,
September 22, 1975

The headstones—a gift from a Valdosta, Georgia merchant named Oscar Cohen—had Shalom inscribed at the bottom. Rachel looked around and found two stones. She placed one on each of the graves.

They walked to the road, where Clete was waiting in the car to take Sammy and his parents to the Kaminsky's house. Frieda and Nathan were going to stay there for the three days of shiva. For the first time other than a Jewish holiday, Lansky's Market was closed.

Since they were the bereaved, the Lanskys were the first to sit for lunch, and, after they began to eat, Mrs. Kaminsky put out a spread of traditional Jewish and Southern foods. It was as if Minsk had moved to Mayberry, with Jews eating collard greens and Southern goyim eating bagels and lox.

"Rachel," Sammy said, taking a bite of hard-boiled egg. "You were right about everything. That's how all this happened . . ." he stopped in mid-sentence.

She held him in her arms and kissed his cheek. Sammy kissed her, then picked up a napkin and wiped his eyes. "I'm going back to Cordele with Clete to get my car and take care of a few of Buddy's things. I want to talk to you when I get back."

Rachel studied him. "You can't be serious! Going back to Cordele? The police reports I heard said the guys that killed Buddy had gotten away—that they might be around here. You can't be on the road by yourself. It's too dangerous."

Sammy shook his head. "No. It's not," he said, looking directly at her without expression.

◆ ◆ ◆

THE SCUTTLEBUTT AT TOMMY'S BARBER SHOP IN CORDELE was that a citizen's manhunt was being organized to track down these criminals before "the folks of Crisp County get to be just as scared to sleep at night as those people in Atlanta." Rumor had it that the sheriff of nearby Ben Hill County had volunteered his champion bloodhounds for the task.

Perkins' Ace Hardware sold out of shotgun shells and home alarm systems within an hour of opening on Monday. The chief of police appealed for calm, saying that a full investigation was underway. The *Cordele Dispatch* was a daily afternoon paper, so by the time it ran the story, the town was in a frenzy. Johnny Underwood, as the officer on duty at the time of the crime, was interviewed and said no composites would be available because the murderers had been masked. The only witness who had seen anything was Buddy Ambrose and, before he died, he said the boys had taken off after a skirmish. Underwood was interviewed on the five o'clock news out of Macon and said, "The perpetrators wore stockings on their faces and were probably some boys from Mexico looking for money to buy drugs. They may be aloose somewhere out of state by now."

◆ ◆ ◆

WHILE THE CITIZENS OF CORDELE ORGANIZED A MANHUNT and a small group sat shiva in Fitzgerald, a few of Big Boy Bates' friends had gathered at his house in Arabi—halfway between the two towns.

Monroe Jarvis, retired chief of police in Cordele, handed a glass of water to Monas and signaled for him to drink. He dialed a number, and as it rang he said, "Now you say what I told you to—okay now, boy?" With that, he put the phone up to Monas' mouth.

"Mr. Dole, this is Monas." Three rapid-fire tics in a row ensued before he spoke again. "Sorry we've been out of touch for a couple of days."

"Well, what happened?"

"Mission accomplished, Mr. Dole." He hesitated for a second, causing Big Boy to nudge him and motion for him to continue. "They ain't going to talk. Neither is their son."

"Good, good. Where are you boys?"

"Laying low in . . ." He looked at his captor. "We're, uh, in Florida. We, uh, need to, uh . . ." Monas hesitated. Monroe shoved a piece of paper in his face, held Monas' head still, and pointed to the line that his captive was to say next: "We need to stay put for a few more days, uh, just in case, you know."

"Sure, sure," Dellwood answered. "Listen, any sign of our buddy, Sam?"

"None," Monas replied.

"Okay. You guys check back in a few days."

Monroe gave Monas the sign to put the phone down. "Good job," Monroe said, pinching Monas on the cheek. "Now you boys run off with Big Boy here and remember: Behave yourselves."

Big Boy had chains around the men's legs and hands and a rope around their necks and, except when Monas had talked to Dellwood, they had duct tape covering their mouths. They had on their fancy suit pants, and that was it. Their faces and torsos were so swollen, they looked like one huge blister. The only man-made wounds they had came from their skirmish with Buddy. The bugs of South Georgia, worse than any biblical plague, had feasted on their skin.

"C'mon now, boys," Big Boy said. "You been outside too long, all this here fresh air is bad for you." Bates pulled on the ropes and led the men outside to his van.

◆ ◆ ◆

AFTER SEVERAL HOURS AT THE KAMINSKYS', Clete, Rayann and Sammy were ready to leave. Sammy kissed his parents, saying he would be at their house and would return the next afternoon. Rachel walked with Sammy to the car.

"So, when you get back, you *are* going to tell me what all of this is about? I mean, your parents have been beaten, Buddy's dead, the killers escaped, and . . . "

Sammy put his arm around her. "Like I said, you were right about Dole and Morton . . . and Mo. Only problem is, you were more right than you know."

"What do you mean?" Rachel asked.

Sammy and Rachel got to the car. Rayann motioned for Clete to get behind the wheel and let Sammy and Rachel talk.

"They sucked me in," he said, standing by the passenger door. "And when I found out, they threatened my parents to keep me quiet."

"Oh, my God," she said, closing her eyes and touching Sammy's face with her trembling fingers.

Sammy hugged her. "We'll talk when I come back." He kissed her, got in the car, and rolled down the window. She bent down so that they were close. "I'll see you tomorrow. I love you."

Rachel said nothing, and the car drove away.

As they moved off toward Cordele, Clete told his wife, "Honey, Sammy and I been friends for a long time. We got some things to discuss that's private. Just drop me off at Mama and Papa L's. Sammy'll bring me home."

Rayann turned toward Clete in the passenger seat. "This doesn't have anything to do with the two boys the police are looking for, does it?" she asked knowingly.

"Hell, no," said Clete. "Those boys are armed and dangerous killers. I'm a businessman, not a vigilante." He looked over his shoulder at Sammy in the back seat. "Sammy here is a man of healing. He don't need to get involved with no po-lice work."

"Neither do you, Cletis Towns," Rayann snapped. "You let the police handle this matter—that's what they're paid for."

Clete shrugged his shoulders. "Okay, okay. Believe me, I ain't getting into the crime business."

When they arrived at Frieda and Nathan's house, Sammy got out, and Clete leaned toward Rayann. "See you in a little while, honey. Sammy just needs some comforting."

She stared at Clete, then kissed his lips. "Don't let your love for Sammy and his family make you do something you might be ashamed of."

"I won't," Clete said, straightening up. "Believe me, that's one thing that ain't gonna happen. I ain't gonna do nothin' I'd be ashamed of."

He and Sammy went into the house. They took off their suit coats and sat down in the kitchen. "Sammy," Clete said, looking at his watch. "I know it's only three o'clock in the afternoon, but since I ain't working today, I think I'll be on an international schedule." He looked at the refrigerator. "It's after five somewhere—I'm gonna get me something to drink."

Sammy, who had been very quiet, nodded. Clete opened the refrigerator, looked around, and the only thing he could find was some Manischewitz wine. He poured two glasses. He and Sammy drank in silence, both grimacing when the sickeningly sweet liquid hit their throats. Sammy twirled the remaining liquid in his glass and said, "You think it's time?"

Clete took a swallow and nodded. They left the wine on the table and went into the den to use the phone. Sammy took a pile of cards out of his wallet, stopping when he got to the right one. He picked up the receiver and took a deep breath. His heart was pounding furiously. He tried to dial the number, but his shaking hand put the receiver in its cradle. Wiping sweat from his face, he put his hand back on the receiver but did not pick it up this time. He stared at Clete sitting across from him.

"Do it for Buddy," Clete said. "He was a man of God, and the Bible says an eye for an eye. We ain't gonna harm nobody, just teach 'em a lesson." Clete picked up the phone and handed it to Sammy, who held it until the dial tone changed, then put it back down.

I would've killed the SS officer, Sammy thought. *I would've enjoyed it even though he was my father.* He picked up the phone, looked at the card one more time, and called.

"Dellwood Dole," the velvety voice said.

"You win, you slimy SOB," Sammy said with a menacing voice.

There was silence on the other end of the phone for a second, then Dellwood said, "Sam! How good to hear your little cracker voice."

"Asshole," Sammy whispered.

"Oh, now, Sam. It wasn't me that screwed things up. You could've been a millionaire many times over if you'd kept your damn mouth shut."

Sammy took a deep breath. "I'm finished with you guys. You leave my parents and me alone, and I'll keep quiet."

"Just like that, my dear, young Sam?" Dellwood said with a chuckle. "No fight? No legal battles lead by your friend Hamburger or that other clown—what was his name? Kessler?"

Sammy did not reply.

"Well, so much for a beautiful relationship," Dellwood said finally. "We do have some papers you'll need to sign—resigning from the board, that sort of thing. Shall we courier them to you?"

Sammy looked up at Clete and smiled. He gave his friend the high sign. "And deny me the chance to tell you in person what a slimy asshole you are?" Sammy said. "No way."

"Hmmm," Dellwood replied. "You want to meet at Mo's or what?"

"Nope." Sammy nodded to Clete.

"Where then, pray tell?" Dellwood seemed less cocksure.

"Here, my parents' house."

Dellwood jeered, "Good luck, Sam. I get hives whenever I leave Atlanta and venture into the hinterlands."

"Well, Dell, old boy—or is it Woody?" Sammy's tone was a mocking one. "You'd better take some Benadryl cause I'm not leaving here. I'm safe here, and if you don't bring those papers to me—" He paused for a second to laugh. "Then I'll take this to the D.A.'s office in Atlanta."

Clete handed Sammy a small tape recorder, which he flipped to the "on" position, and Dellwood was treated to his confession.

"Where the hell!" Dellwood screamed. "How'd you get. . . ? You bastard! You taped it."

"How perceptive, my dear Dell." Sammy turned off the tape. He smiled at Clete, who sat on the sofa and grinned. "This," Sammy said, kissing the tape player, "is my insurance policy."

"How do I know you won't use it even if I come down there?" Dellwood spoke in measured tones.

"Well, I'll tell you." Sammy took a seat by the phone. "You don't. But, if you leave me alone for the rest of my life," he advised, leaning back in his chair, "then I'll do the same. If you bother me or my parents, this tape will come out of hiding. We have to trust each other and, after all, if you can't trust your good friends, then who can you trust, huh? Capisce, my dear little Dell?"

"You goddamn bastard," Dellwood yelled. "You're out of your league, Lansky. You're a bush leaguer trying to play with the big boys."

Clete had poured them each another glass of wine. Sammy nodded and took a sip. "You're absolutely right. I don't even want to be one of the big boys. You and I both want the same thing—to get me out of the deal completely—forget I was ever in it."

Dellwood was silent.

"I'll sign your papers," Sammy said, "if you personally bring them to me, and then promise to get out of here immediately after the ink's dry and never come back. You forget you ever knew me, and I'll pretend this has all been a bad dream, which it has been."

After a moment of silence, Dellwood began to laugh. "What? You mean, your parents aren't going to have us over for lunch? We thought they were so hospitable, particularly after the way they welcomed Monas and Steele into their home." Dellwood laughed harder, and his tone became more caustic. "I was hoping to stop by and have some of that food you kikes eat."

"I sign, you leave."

"Okay, okay," Dellwood said in mock seriousness. "If you want to be so antisocial, be that way. Henry and I will be there around noon tomorrow. Oh, and by the way, Sam, we'll be bringing along some boys that make Monas and Steele look like Harvard grads. So don't let your hormones get uppity. Get my drift?"

Sammy grunted.

"Bye-bye, Sam," said Dellwood, laughing as the phone clicked in Sammy's ear.

Sammy put the phone down, took a deep breath, looked at Clete for a second, and said, "We're on."

CHAPTER SEVENTEEN 17

BY ELEVEN O'CLOCK TUESDAY MORNING, Sammy was pacing. He had begun in the kitchen and continued the vigil in his parents' living room. With its position at the front of the house and two windows looking out onto the street, the living room was a perfect place to wait and watch for Dellwood and his henchmen. Finally, at 12:30, he saw a large black Lincoln roll past the house, stop for a second, then back up and enter the driveway. He walked from the small living room toward the kitchen but stopped short when he heard a car door slam. Sweat began to drip down his face and onto his torso as he waited.

The screen door opened, and a stocky, bald man with a thick neck and upper body entered. He was swarthy and had low-set, small ears and an S-shaped nose. He pushed back the screen door, took one look at Sammy, and rushed toward him. Before Sammy could raise his arms in defense, the man had grabbed him and twisted one of his arms behind his back. Sammy moaned with pain but stopped when a second man—tall, thin, and pockmarked, with large dark eyebrows hanging over sinister eyes—grabbed him by the throat and held pressure. Pockmarked smelled of stale cigarettes.

Dellwood, dressed casually in black pants, a royal blue silk shirt and a black and hunter green argyle cashmere sweater vest, walked in with Henry not far behind.

"So good to see you, Sam," Dellwood said. "Sorry we have to meet under such circumstances. He turned to the two goons who had Sammy wrapped up. "Take him," he said, making a motion with his fingers, "in there." He pointed above their heads toward the living room.

The men pushed Sammy into the living room, threw him into a wing chair, and quickly bound his hands and feet with rope. Dellwood and Henry followed. Henry sat, but before Dellwood did the same, he walked slowly over to the curtains, found a pull cord behind one of them, closed them, then sank into the plastic-covered sofa.

"What is this shit?" he demanded. "Jesus H. Christ! With all the money we paid you, the least you could've done was buy your parents some new furniture. What kind of a son are you, Sam?" Dellwood got up and walked to a tattered print chair.

"Henry, the papers." He extended his hand toward his partner without looking at him. "We'll let Sam here have his right hand free in a moment to sign." Henry produced the papers from his briefcase and pushed them toward Sammy.

Just as the stockier of the two goons started to free his right hand to sign, Sammy began to laugh and in a loud voice, sang out: "Welcome aboard! It's the Chattanooga Choo-Choo, track forty-nine . . ."

"What the hell's wrong with you?" yelled Dole. "Shut up. Stuff something in his goddamn mouth."

Pockmarked fumbled around in his back pocket and found a greasy handkerchief, which he began to stuff into Sammy's mouth. Sammy clenched down on the man's fingers as hard as he could, causing Pockmarked to let out a mighty scream. The man cradled his fingers, yelled, and fell at Sammy's feet. He was still whimpering and gyrating when his stocky partner lunged toward Sammy with a fist. The blow fell short as Clete, who had been hiding in the small living room closet, grabbed the man's arms and pulled back, grunting furiously as he did. Another man stepped from the closet and threw a thick rope around Swarthy's neck, forcing him to forget his fight with Clete and try to free his neck from the rope. Clete took an electric cord from his pocket and began to wrap it around the man's legs. Swarthy kicked backward, hitting Clete squarely in the groin. Clete screamed, then he tackled the man's legs in a frenzy. All three combatants fell to the floor.

Swarthy, the rope still tightening around his neck, turned toward Clete and swung, hitting him in the jaw. Clete released a series of blows to the man's face, but they had little effect. The three of them, arms and legs flailing in every direction, rolled around in a ball. Dole and Henry watched, frozen. Pockmarked, whose finger had been filleted to the bone, lay in front of them, screaming.

Monroe Jarvis and a few of his buddies poured into the room from various hiding places in the den. Stewball Barnes crept up behind the bitten man and dented his skull with a lead pipe, rendering him unconscious. Barnes followed the other three men around the room until he caught Clete's eye. When they saw each other, Clete moved away from the fray for a second and gave Stewball a clear shot. The pipe landed squarely on Swarthy's forehead, and the battle was over. Sammy was freed, and he and two others tied Henry's and Dellwood's hands and duct taped their mouths. The unconscious goons were tied up and taped.

A few of Sammy's buddies from high school walked in, each of them carrying an old, bald, clay-stained automobile tire. Dellwood's eyes bulged, and he squirmed furiously as he watched the tires being placed—one by one—over the unconscious men's heads and down onto and around their arms. Dellwood shook, seizure-like, when the tire was put over Henry's head and muffled screams emanated from inside his duct tape when his turn came.

Sammy, rubbing his wrists to take the sting out, began to pace around the room. He stopped, putting his nose in the air and sniffing.

"Damn," he said, looking at Clete. "Something die in here? Smells like someone is rotting from the inside."

Clete held his nose and pointed toward Dellwood. Sammy looked at the bound man and grabbed him by the shoulder, turning him sideways just a bit. He sniffed and shook his head. "I wonder if shit stains Armani pants?" He pointed toward Dellwood's seat from which a putrid brown liquid oozed. "Anybody know?" he asked, looking around the room. Several of the men shook their heads.

Sammy proceeded to pace in front of Dole, as if preparing for a jury summation. The only sound was the whimpering of the captured. He stopped, moved the back of a small chair right in front of Dellwood and sat down, folding his arms across the chair and leaning forward, directly in Dellwood's face. Scrunching up his nose, he said in a low voice, "Damn, Dellwood, what the hell you been eating?" Sammy backed his chair up, away from the odor, then stood up, walked around the chair, grabbed Dole's neck and lifted him off the sofa—he was eyeball to eyeball with his adversary.

"Nobody," he said through clenched teeth, "nobody, fucks with my family. A lot of people have tried—people who make you guys look like choirboys—but nobody does it with me around." He released Dellwood, who fell back on the sofa.

"You boys figured you'd come down here and scare me," Sammy said as he sat back down. "We sort of turned the tables on you, didn't we? Now, when the urge to get nasty comes over you in the future, I want you to remember what happened here today and think about it real hard." He opened his arms and turned around to look at his friends. "Cause these boys don't give too many folks a second chance. Oh, and the other thing. I'm going to resign from the management all right; don't worry about that. But, in the future, that is if you boys want to have a future, the doctors are going to own ninety-five percent of the machine, and you pukes own five percent. Pretty generous of the doctors, if you ask me, since they paid for it in the first place."

"Sammy, Sammy! Where are you, boy?" a voice called from the direction of the kitchen.

"Living room," Sammy yelled back.

Big Boy Bates, dressed in overalls, entered, smiled broadly, and spit a wad of tobacco into a Styrofoam cup. "Got a delivery for you, son," he said.

"Good timing," Sammy replied, taking a few steps toward Big Boy.

Big Boy whistled, and his brother-in-law walked in dragging two metal chains. Attached to the chains by the neck, hands, and feet were Monas and Steele. There was no tape covering their mouths, but they said nothing. At the sight of this, Dellwood vomited, the noxious fluid pouring out over the duct tape onto his cashmere sweater.

Monroe Jarvis walked up to Sammy, put his massive arm around the younger man's shoulder, and guided him into the den. He spoke to Sammy in a soft but strong voice.

"You go on down to Fitzgerald now, son. You got business down there that's a lot more important than this we got going here." Monroe looked toward the living room when he spoke the last few words.

"But. . . ," Sammy said.

Monroe squeezed Sammy's arm. "Go on now, son." He stared at Sammy for a second, then pushed the younger man through the kitchen and out the screen door into the carport. Monroe let go of Sammy's arm and stepped up on the stoop leading into the kitchen.

He looked at Sammy and said with no expression, "See you later. You get outta here now. Your job is done."

Sammy watched the large man close the screen door and disappear into the kitchen. Since his car was parked on the street, Sammy started to walk in that direction, but his removal from the scene just didn't sit right, so he stopped and returned to the carport. He waited outside the screen door for a moment, then gingerly pried it open. He could hear Monroe's booming voice.

"Boys, first I want to apologize to you. Here we are tusslin' with each other, and we ain't even been formally introduced." He looked around the room and waved. "My name is Monroe Jarvis, and until just recently, I was the chief of po-lice here in Cordele."

Sammy heard nothing for a moment. He crept a few steps into the kitchen. Monroe continued. "It just hit me that you boys may not even realize that we, all of us, are in Cordele as we speak. Welcome to Cordele, boys! Anyway, we got a funny habit down here of taking care of our own. This is our home, and we just don't take too well to some city boys like y'all coming into our home uninvited."

Sammy heard nothing but muffled tones for a few seconds, then Monroe raised his voice. "In particular, we take exception to you boys just showing up, beating up two of our finest citizens, and killing another.

"I guess you boys told someone you was coming down here, but the way I got it figured, something must've happened to you. No one ever saw any of you." Sammy felt flushed. He crept a little closer, and his heart was racing. He had no idea what Monroe was going to say.

"Oh, sure, they'll be an investigation and all, but after a while, with no leads, things'll settle back to normal. Po-lice work, particularly missing persons investigations, tends to be that way. If you don't find them soon, people forget about the poor missing persons." He paused for a second. "Course, here we got us a small force, so with a manhunt for them murderers going on full speed, I doubt we got much of a chance of finding a few boys what was headed to Cordele and never made it. In fact, you know what, Big Boy?"

Sammy could barely hear the response. "What, Mon-roe?"

"I been sitting in courtrooms watching slick lawyers get slime balls like this off for years. I think we're doing a civic duty by saving the taxpayers a lot of money. I mean, trials are expensive."

Sammy heard Big Boy's unmistakable cackle, then Big Boy said, "Yeah, good thing we ain't got no records on these fellas. Might have to burn the courthouse down like they did in the old days."

Monroe laughed, then his voice rose with a serious tone. "Now I'm gonna tell you how your last day on Earth is gonna be spent."

Whoa, what was he talking about? Sammy thought. They had lured Dellwood and company down here to scare the hell out of them. That's all he'd signed on for.

Monroe spoke. "Yesterday, I went to Buddy's funeral and heard the preacher talking about how they was putting Buddy's body in the ground, but his soul was on its way to heaven and that our prayers could help it get there. Well, boys, all of us here is gonna be praying for you, too—only we ain't trying to help your souls go to heaven. We just want you to be closer to your final destination."

Sammy scrunched up his face in confusion. *What was going on? Was Monroe serious, or was this just more scare tactics?*

"Buddy built a fall-out shelter about fifteen years ago. Built it underground about ten feet—figured he'd survive a nuclear attack, then be ready to fight the Commies, I guess. He was crazy, but that was Buddy. Anyway, it's got a few basic necessities, not much. In fact, if you want to know about the accommodations, why don't you ask these two with the chains around their necks. They been down there for a couple of days."

Oh, shit! They told me Big Boy had them locked up in his basement, Sammy thought.

There was silence. Sammy could hear some rustling around and what sounded like whimpering. "Now, you may be asking yourselves how long you gonna be down there?" Monroe said. "Well don't fret boys, you're gonna be there less than twenty-four hours." Monroe paused again. "Because, before he was *murdered,* Buddy sold the land around and on top of the shelter to Ogelthorpe Power to enlarge Lake Blackshear. They been clear-cutting the place like crazy for months. And . . . at six tomorrow morning, they gonna flood the land with you pukes *in* the shelter. So, all of a sudden, instead of ten feet down, you're gonna be about thirty feet down." Monroe began to yell, "And when that water covers that shelter and you take your last gasp of air, then *your* souls will be going straight to HELL!"

Sammy burst into the living room and screamed at Monroe. "No way! No, one murder's enough." He looked around the room and found Clete. "Clete, we can't do this." Tears streamed down Sammy's cheeks, and his voice cracked. His eyes pleaded with Clete first, then Monroe. "It's wrong, completely wrong . . ."

Clete looked Sammy straight in the eye. "Nothing could be more right, Sammy," he said. "With these boys alive, you got no security."

"No!" Sammy screamed loud enough so that all eyes turned to him and there was silence. "There have been enough murders, enough killing. No more."

"Only one so far, Sammy," Monroe said. "But we're aiming to avenge that one with a few more."

Sammy shook his head and said over and over, "No more. No more killing."

Monroe and Bates grabbed Sammy by the arms and tried to pull him back to the carport. "You ain't never seen or heard nothin' about no boys from Atlanta," Big Boy said, glaring at Sammy. "Now git."

Sammy had been friends with Big Boy since childhood, but that didn't prevent him from punching his friend squarely on the jaw. Big Boy backed up with an astonished look on his face, holding his cheek. Sammy glared at his friend. "I said there will be no more killing." They stared at each other for a second, then Sammy turned toward Dellwood.

"I have this tape." He took the tape out of his pants pocket and held it in the air. "And both Kessler and Hamburger have a copy of it. Any more trouble and the tape goes to the D.A., and you boys go to hell."

There was silence for a moment. Monroe shook his head. "Sammy, son, you may live to regret this here decision."

Sammy patted his old friend on the shoulder. "No, I won't, Monroe. This is the only way it can be."

All of the captured, except Monas and Steele, were handcuffed, then had their ropes removed. When it came time to unhook Buddy's murderers from their chains, Sammy and Bates stared at each other. Sammy took a deep breath, then nodded. Bates pulled on their chains and said, "C'mon boys, you got a date with Lucifer." He walked toward his van dragging the half-dead Monas and Steele behind him.

Henry Morton was untied and put into the driver's seat. The goons, still woozy, were stuffed into the back seat and forced to lie on top of each other. They removed the tape from Dellwood's mouth, but he still wore the cuffs just like the others. When they were out of sight, Sammy hugged his friends and whispered,

"Thanks. Thanks for taking care of me and Buddy. Thanks for stopping when I asked you to."

Clete chuckled. "Aw, hell, we weren't gonna kill the bastards. We was just gonna give 'em a few hours down in the shelter to think about mending their ways. Let 'em know what might happen to 'em if they was to come back down in these parts for any reason other than passing through on the way to Florida."

Sammy looked at his friend, who had a grin on his face.

Clete continued. "Can you imagine what they'd a thought after a hour or two down there just waiting for the water to cover their sorry asses?"

Monroe Jarvis put his arm on Clete's shoulder. "Yeah, I'd hate to be the dry cleaner that got them pairs of britches."

They all smiled.

◆ ◆ ◆

SAMMY DROVE TO FITZGERALD, HIS MOUTH DRY, HIS PULSE RACING, his nerves stretched to the maximum and ready to snap. Every Yom Kippur, Rabbi Kohen had said, "A righteous man lives on after his death; the wicked are dead even while they are alive." He could have let his friends kill Dellwood and company, for they were so wicked they had died inside long ago. But just as his father hadn't been able to kill the Nazi years before, he couldn't let his friends kill now. As he drove, Sammy was sure of only one thing—finally, Gottfried Heydrich was dead.

CHAPTER EIGHTEEN 18

Sammy stopped at the Race Trac gas station on the outskirts of Fitzgerald to clean up, then drove to the Kaminskys'. There were three cars on the street outside the house, and he parked behind one.

"Sammy, good to see you," said Mrs. Kaminsky in a Southern drawl. "Your mama and papa been wondering when you were going to get here."

Sammy smiled at her, then went to greet his parents, who were sitting with Rachel on an ornate couch in the Kaminskys' large living room.

"Sweetheart, how are you?" his mother asked, rising to kiss him.

"Doing all right, doing all right," Sammy said as he hugged her. He leaned over to kiss his father and Rachel. Rachel stood and wrapped her arms around his neck.

"Everything okay?" she whispered.

"Yeah."

Rachel released her arms from his neck and looked at his face. "Any news about Buddy's killers?"

He kissed Rachel and brought her close to him. "Everything is okay," he whispered.

She squeezed him and said, "You always say that but never mean it." She stepped back a foot. "I need you. My life is incomplete without you."

"Sit, Sammy, sit," said Mrs. Kaminsky, taking him from Rachel. "Have some lunch, have a snack, we've got enough here for days. Look," she said, pointing into the dining room. "We got cold cuts, cakes, a fruit tray, a Jell-O mold . . ." She looked at her watch. "And if you're here for another hour or so, Sonya Moscowitz is bringing a baked chicken."

"Thanks," Sammy replied, sitting down across from his parents. They looked drawn and tired, but there was still a gleam in their eyes that assured Sammy of their incredible resilience.

"So, everything is okay at home?" Nathan asked.

Sammy nodded.

"Oh, before I forget, please water the plants in the kitchen," Frieda said. "Not too much, now, maybe once while we're here."

Sammy nodded again. He smiled inwardly.

"Any news about the killers?" asked Frieda.

"Nope," Sammy replied.

Nathan leaned over to his wife and kissed her. "They won't be back. Our police are too smart for them."

Frieda shook her head and looked worried. "In the old country, they used to say that a murderer always returns to the scene of his crime."

"That's in movies and on TV, Mama," Sammy said.

"Everything what is in the movies happens in real life," Frieda said, waving her finger at him. "Where you think those big-shot directors they get their ideas, huh? Trust me on that, Schmuel. I had an aunt in Poland who used to say that the spirit of the victim lures the killer back to the scene of the crime."

"What nonsense," Nathan said, looking at Sammy and shaking his head. "Was that the same aunt who put the chicken bone above the mezuzah to make sure the Angel of Death would pass over the house? What a meshuggenah."

Frieda cut him a look. "We are in a house of mourning for a man we raised as our son. Don't use that kind of word in such a house."

Nathan looked at Sammy and said in a soft voice, "Your mother, she has told me before that this aunt was meshug . . . crazy."

"Umm," said Frieda leaning toward her husband so she wouldn't miss his comment. "Well, I'm telling you that what she said about the spirit of the victim luring the killer is true."

Nathan patted her hands. "Don't worry. Mr. Perkins has a shotgun reserved for me, *and* he's going to show me how to use it."

"Oiy, gevald!" Frieda threw her arms in the air. There were only four people there, but they turned to look at her when she shouted, so she lowered her voice. "They kill Buddy, then you kill yourself trying to kill them. You, who haven't touched a gun in forty years. I ask you, who's meshuggenah?"

Nathan spoke directly to Sammy. "In Bialystok, the SS, they came into my house, beat me, and took away my life. I will make my last stand here. Anyone who comes into my house, like the SS, will get what we should have given them."

"Oiy!" said Frieda. She got off the sofa, and walked over to a friend.

Sammy rubbed his father's hand and leaned over to kiss him. He walked to the table, but, even though he had not eaten in over twenty-four hours, the shock of the day's events dulled his appetite. He put some food on his plate but only picked at it. Rachel came up to him, rubbed his shoulder, and spoke, "When are we going to talk?" she asked.

Sammy moved some fruit around on his plate. "How about now?"

She nodded. Mrs. Kaminsky approached. Rachel grabbed Sammy's hand and said, "Let's walk."

He laid his plate down and they went out into the late afternoon sun. Rachel put her arm in his as they strolled toward downtown. "So?" she asked.

Sammy took a deep breath, then told her about how Dellwood and his buddies had stolen the money. He admitted that her suspicions had lingered with him and told her about how he'd caught them tapping his phone. He told her about his meeting at Mo's, his escape from them, about staying at Buddy's and how Buddy had died protecting his parents.

"When I first saw Buddy at the house, he was alive. I checked on Mama and Papa, and when I came back, it looked to me like he was just resting, but when I got close to him—" Sammy stopped and wiped a tear from his eye. "The bullet must've hit his superior vena cava or his subclavian. He never had a chance."

They walked in silence for a moment. "What happens next?" Rachel asked. "I'm assuming your good friend Mo is in the middle of this whole thing."

Sammy nodded. "You were right about him, too." He took a deep breath. "I'm finished with him. Maybe I'll talk to the guys in Albany about a job, maybe . . ." He took her hand and squeezed it. "Maybe I found the missing colors and you'll come back."

Rachel stopped walking in front of the old Masonic Hall, turned and faced him. "I love you, Sammy, and nothing would make me happier. But what about Dellwood and his crowd? You said yourself they'd fixed it so it would appear that you had stolen all the money." She took Sammy's hand. "These guys are out of your league, Sammy. They'll be after you next." They approached Lee Street and the synagogue.

"Let's sit for a moment," he said. They sat on the sun-baked steps of the synagogue, surrounded by the huge hydrangeas the congregation had planted a lifetime ago. It was too early for blooms, but in this warm climate, large leaves filled the stalks with green.

Sammy squinted. "Dellwood and company aren't going to bother me."

Rachel shook her head. "Ah, c'mon, Sammy. You're being incredibly naïve."

A station wagon stopped in front of the synagogue, and a load of children dashed out of the car, onto the steps, and into the building. Sammy and Rachel recognized the driver and waved as she pulled away.

"I've made a deal with them." He covered his forehead with his hand. "They leave me alone, and I leave them alone."

Rachel bolted up and stood above him. "What?! Are you nuts?" She shook her head and looked heavenward. "They'll blackmail you for the rest of your life." She leaned over and grabbed his arm. "And even if they don't, what happens if this little scheme gets uncovered?" She sat down and lifted his chin with her hand. "You need to go to the police right away. Tell them the truth. That way, it's your word against theirs. Otherwise, *you* may end up in jail."

He removed her hand from his chin and kissed it. He then told Rachel of the events of the past few hours.

"This is crazy." Her voice cracked, and Sammy noticed that she was trembling. "You're their prisoner—for life. You'll have to watch your back everywhere you go."

Sammy shook his head and took a small cassette out of his front pocket. "This," he said, waving it in front of her, "is my insurance policy."

She furrowed her brow and reached for the tape. He put it back in his pocket. "I had a tape recorder hidden in my underwear at Mo's. I taped Dellwood telling me exactly how they had set the whole thing up—it amounts to a confession. When I played this over the phone for Dellwood, we came to an understanding of sorts. That's why he was willing to come down here for me to sign his papers. I'm through with him and he with me. With the welcome reception we gave them, I'll bet they won't be heading this way anytime in the next fifty years."

Rachel rubbed her hands through her hair and sighed. "And Buddy's killers?"

Sammy took a deep breath. "Big Boy took them away."

Rachel stared at him.

The cantor rushed by, stepping to the side of them. "End of the year program—we've got to practice," he said in passing as he entered the synagogue. They nodded and smiled at him.

Singing echoed inside the building behind them. Sammy and Rachel listened in silence for a moment, after which he stood, stretched, and shielded his eyes from the sun. He took her by the hand, and together they entered the small sanctuary and sat in a back pew. He put his arm around her shoulder.

"I have someone I want you to meet," he whispered.

She put her head on his arm. "Who?"

Sammy said nothing. He closed his eyes and listened to the music. The youngsters, under the direction of the cantor, were in great voice as they sang a tune Sammy remembered from his childhood:

"Henai matov uma n'ayim shevat achim gam yachad."

"How wonderful it will be to dwell with our brothers again."

ABOUT THE AUTHOR

CHARLES GERSHON was born and reared in Atlanta, Georgia. He received his bachelor's degree from the University of Pennsylvania and an M.D. from Emory University, where he graduated magna cum laude. He completed his post-graduate training in urological surgery at the University of Michigan. He lives in Asheville, North Carolina with his wife and two children. This is his first novel.